COLLECTION
Apparented lasers and technologies

Coordination: Serge Dahan, Bertrand Pusel

Facial Rejuvenation

Lasers, lights and energy based devices

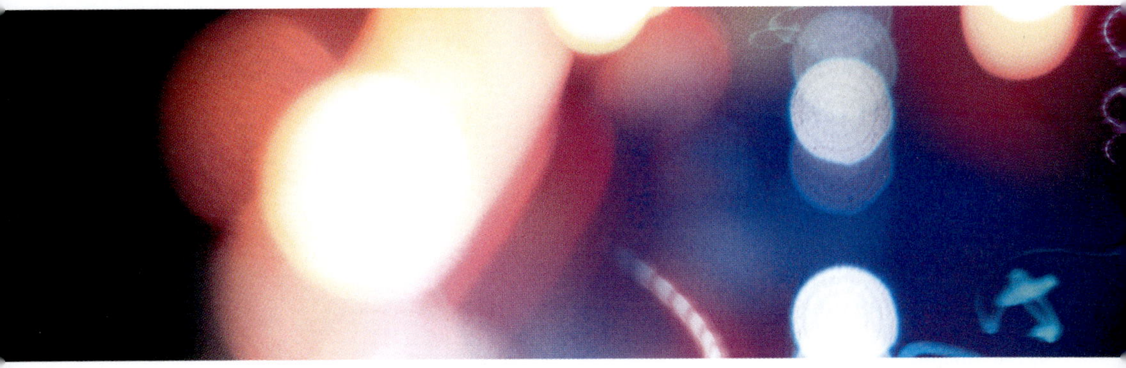

doin

In the “Lasers et technologies apparentées” collection, éditions Doin

Erythro-couperose et rosacée, coordination: Serge Dahan, Bertrand Pusel, 2012
La photothérapie dynamique, coordination: Serge Dahan, Bertrand Pusel, 2014
Rajeunissement du visage, coordination: Serge Dahan, Bertrand Pusel, 2014
Photobiomodulation en dermatologie, coordination: Serge Dahan, Bertrand Pusel, Hugues Cartier, 2014

In the “Dermatologie pratique” collection, éditions Doin

Les lasers en dermatologie, 3e édition, coordination: Hugues Cartier, Serge Dahan, Gérard Toubel, 2011

Doin éditeurs

Éditions John Libbey Eurotext
127, avenue de la République
92120 Montrouge

John Libbey Eurotext Limited
42-46 High Street
Esher
KT109QY
United Kingdom

ISBN: 978-2-7040-1414-9

List of authors

Ascher Benjamin
11, rue Fresnel
75116 Paris – France

Avram Mathew
MGH Dermatology Laser
& Cosmetic Center
Massachusetts General Hospital
Harvard Medical School
50, Staniford Street
Boston, MA 02114 – USA

Badawi Ashraf
National Institute
of Laser Enhanced Sciences
Université du Caire Oula
Giza – Egypt

Bassi Andrea
Section of Dermatology
Department of Critical Care Medicine
and Surgery
University of Florence
Villa S. Chiara
Piazza Indipendenza 11
50129 Florence – Italy

Benzekri Laila
Centre hospitalo-universitaire Ibn Sina
Service de dermatologie
Rue Famfdal Cherkaoui Rabat Instituts
Rabat – Morocco

Bonan Paolo
Laser Dermatology
Donatello Surgery Clinic
Villa Donatello
Piazzale Donatello 14
50132 Florence – Italy

Bruscino Nicola
Department of Surgery
and Translational Medicine
Section of Dermatology, University
of Florence
Viale Michelangelo 41
50129 Florence – Italy

Cartier Hugues
Centre médical Saint-Jean
8, square Saint-Jean
62000 Arras – France

Conti Rossana
Section of Dermatology
Department of Critical Care Medicine
and Surgery
University of Florence
Villa S. Chiara
Piazza Indipendenza 11
50129 Florence – Italy

Dahan Serge
Clinique Saint-Jean-Languedoc
20, route de Revel
31077 Toulouse – France

Farsani Terry Taraneh
Harvard Combined Dermatology
Residency Program
Massachusetts General Hospital
Bartlett 616, 55 Fruit St. Boston
MA 02114 – USA

Fritz Klaus
Dermatology and Laser Center
Reduitstraße 13
76829 Landau – Germany

Fusade Thierry
Centre Laser et Dermatologie
chirurgicale et esthétique
23, rue de Saint-Pétersbourg
75008 Paris – France

Laubach Hans
Centre Laser et Dermatologie
chirurgicale et esthétique
23, rue Saint Pétersbourg
75008 Paris – France

Le Pillouer-Prost Anne
Service de Dermatologie
Hôpital Privé Clairval
317, boulevard du Redon
13009 Marseille – France

Mazer Jean-Michel
Centre Laser International de la Peau
85, avenue de la Bourdonnais
75007 Paris – France

Naouri Michael
Cabinet Médical – Centre Laser
4, place Leclerc
94130 Nogent-sur-Marne – France

Ortiz Arisa
University of California San Diego
Division of Dermatology
8899 University Center Ln, Suite 350
San Diego, CA 92122 – USA

Pons-Guiraud Annick
10, boulevard Malesherbes
75008 Paris – France

Pusel Bertrand
Villabianca
18, boulevard Pierre Sauvaigo
06570 Saint-Paul-de-Vence – France

Raimbault Catherine
30, rue des Clercs
57000 Metz – France

Rho Nark-Kyoung
Samsung Medical Center
Sungkyunkwan University
81, Irwon-Ro Gangnam-gu
Seoul 135-710 – Korea

Tiplica George Sorin
Carol Davila University of
Medecine and Pharmacy
8, boulevard Eroii Sanitari
Bucarest 050474 – Romania

Troiano Michela
Laser Dermatology Research
Section of Dermatology
University of Florence
Villa S.Chiara
Piazza Indipendenza 11
50129 Florence – Italy

Vigneron Jean-Luc
Villabianca
718, boulevard Pierre Sauvaigo
06570 Saint-Paul-de-Vence – France

Foreword

Skin aging is a multidimensional problem. Based on an accurate knowledge of skin anatomy and physiology, we can choose from a large variety of therapeutic options like lasers, energy-based devices, injectable products, skin care and cosmeceuticals. Dermatologists, who know the skin layer by layer, provide such treatments, but every therapist has his or her own favourites.

The ideal rejuvenation technique should improve the tension and texture of superficial epidermal layers, tighten subcutaneous tissue, improve skin laxity and remodel the dermis for dermal collagen. *Laser techniques* and other *aesthetic procedures* sometimes overlap in indication and effect, so they either compete with each other or they can be combined for better results and fewer side effects.

This book summarizes an updated knowledge. It was written by authors who work in aesthetic dermatology every day.

Thanks to the support of the French Laser Dermatology Group, the European Society of Laser Dermatology and the company Avène, this knowledge has been made available to you.

Klaus Fritz, MD
Director of Dermatology and laser centers Landau and Kandel (Germany)
Associate University Professor at the University of Medicine
and pharmacy "Carol Davila", Bukarest
Lecturer and Consultant Dermatologist at the university Osnabrueck (D)
and University clinic Bern (Switzerland)
Past President of ESLD (European Society for Laser Dermatology)
Presidentof the German Academy of Dermatology

Introduction

Like all of our organs, the skin undergoes aging. This process is natural and inevitable, although it is also influenced by our lifestyles.

Today, we are expected to have a young and attractive face in order to meet the diktats of "appearance", a modern trend that has been popularised via the media.

Treatments with lasers, lights and energy-based devices (EBD) are the foundation of managing the facial skin aging; this strategy can also be combined with the use of cosmetics, skin peels, dermal filler injections, or other botulinum toxin treatments.

This treatment must, above all, be ethical, and it is essential to obtain the patient's informed consent in order to harmonize their expectations and the possible outcome of the treatment. It must protect the patient from any deviation that could lead to complications or even permanent side effects.

This can not be achieved unless the practitioner has a good understanding of the pathophysiology and clinical signs of skin aging. It is also paramount that the practitioner thoroughly understands the technology and uses it in compliance with good practice.

Lasers, lights and EBD can reduce pigmented lesions and vascular lesions, fine lines and wrinkles, as well as improve texture and tone.

In this work we review the various types of laser, lights and EBD such as Intense Pulsed Light, LED, radiofrequency and ultrasound. We also review cosmetics and injections, and their potential interactions.

The methods used to evaluate the effects of these technologies on the skin will be detailed as will also be some specific points concerning the treatment of Black, Asian or Mediterranean skin.

The publication of this work would not have been possible without the participation of international and French authors who agreed to offer their time and share their knowledge with us.

Thank you to all of these authors for their excellent contributions, dedication, accuracy, and expertise.

We now leave you with this book, passing on our experience, which will allow each one of us to raise questions, to progress, and to offer our patients the best of our practice in laser, lights and EBD.

Serge Dahan, Bertrand Pusel

Summary

CHAPTER 1

Skin aging, pathophysiology and clinical signs

Serge Dahan

INTRODUCTION

Skin aging varies between individuals and is subjected to intricate and cumulative intrinsic factors, specific to each person, as well as to extrinsic factors depending on the individual's lifestyle.

Skin aging needs to be conceptualised in its entirety. It cannot be dissociated from the aging of the adjacent fatty, muscular, and bone structures.

These processes occur in the skin in the same way as in other tissues, and can be described in terms of pathophysiology, histology, and clinical features.

Since it is exposed to public view, the face and its aging can be observed more easily than in other organs. The changes that occur can be quantified using skin-aging scales.

It is only after a thorough clinical examination of the various aspects of facial skin aging that an overall and personalised management plan can be offered, resolving medical as much as aesthetic concerns. This approach to skin aging management should also address the neck, neckline, and hands.

Dermatoporosis is a term introduced in 2004 by J. H. Saurat, in analogy to osteoporosis, and it covers the impacts of chronic cutaneous insufficiency or fragility on the whole of the integumentary system. It must be taken into account in particular when considering the neck, neckline, and hands.

INTRINSIC FACTORS IN SKIN AGING

As we age, all of the body's functions in every organ undergo changes with genetically programmed variations particular to each individual.

Tobacco use, oestrogen deficiency, and menopause are independent risk factors that exacerbate intrinsic skin aging as well as other general illnesses.

Pathophysiology

There are various theories of pathophysiology regarding both genetic mechanisms and the harmful role of free radicals.

In terms of genetics, many genes involved in the aging process have been identified, most of which intervene in stress responses or metabolic activity. For example, the shortening of telomeres points to cell senescence and DNA changes, the activation of p53, and apoptosis.

We also see a reduced ability to fight against oxidative stress with the production of free radicals contributing to intrinsic aging.

Studies have shown that a protein known as MAP (mitogen-activated protein) kinase plays an important role in the regulation of cellular growth factors, the expression of MMP, and the synthesis of procollagen type I.

If this process of regulation is interrupted, there is increased production of matrix metalloproteinases (MMP) leading to collagen degradation affecting MMP 1 (collagenase) and MMP 9 (gelatinase). In addition, blockage of TGF-beta reduces collagen synthesis.

Protein glycation affecting elastin and collagen can also be observed in skin thus weakened.

Histology Fig. 1

With aging, the stratum corneum, which is made of dead cells, thickens. All other components of the skin decrease with aging:

– the epidermis thins, as does the dermoepidermal junction (DEJ);

– there is a reduction of melanocytes (10% every 10 years);

– the DEJ flattens as it is less well maintained, given the deterioration of its supporting fibres (decrease of collagen type IV in the lamina lucida and collagen type VII in the anchoring fibrils).

This DEJ involvement leads to a "loss of connection" between the epidermis and dermis, and subsequently to wrinkles and fine lines;

– the dermis also decreases in thickness with reduced density of collagen and elastic fibres; the vessels are dilated.

After skin rejuvenation using lasers and related technologies, we would hope to achieve improved skin structure, with thickening of the dermis pointing to dermal remodelling and neocollagen formation.

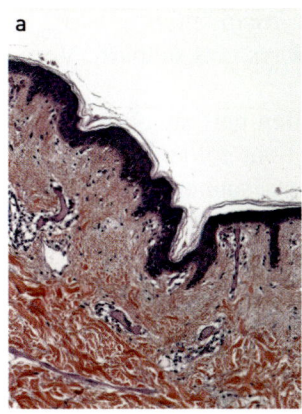

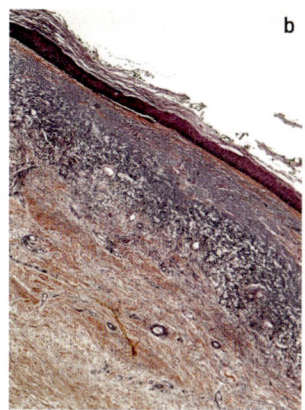

Figure 1 Normal skin (a), aged skin with elastosis and atrophy (b)
(photos Dr Ducoin, Histology – Clinique Saint-Jean Languedoc)

Clinical features

The skin thins, becomes dryer, dehydrated, less elastic, loses tone, and it becomes depigmented with the decrease in secretion of sebum and sweat. It becomes fragile, developing ecchymotic purpura more easily when subject to trauma.

Fine lines and then wrinkles appear first in areas of facial expression and then they become more pronounced, encompassing areas of muscle contraction and those involved in dynamic facial expression.

Using imprints of the skin, the changes in microrelief caused by aging can be demonstrated by the grooves of tiny fine lines that all follow the same direction (anisotropy), in contrast to young skin which shows lines in a number of different directions (isotropy). These imprints are used to evaluate our anti-aging treatments **Fig. 2**.

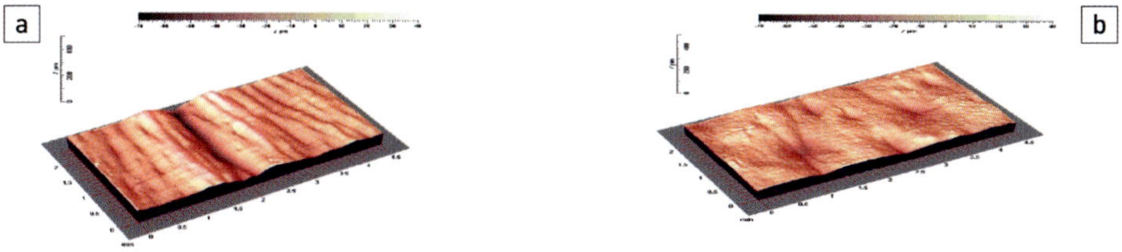

Figure 2 Wrinkle imprints before and after treatment
Before treatment (a), after treatment wrinkles are less prominent (b)

EXTRINSIC FACTORS IN SKIN AGING

Exposure to sunlight, especially when it is repeated and occurs from childhood, will lead to aging of the skin areas exposed to sunlight, all the more so in lighter phototypes; extrinsic aging has some overlap with intrinsic aging.

Phototypes can be categorised using *Fitzpatrick's classification*:

– phototype I: reaction to the sun, does not tan, always gets sunburn. Very fair skin, freckles, blond or red hair;

– phototype II: reaction to the sun, tans poorly, often gets sunburn. Very fair skin, blond or light brown hair, freckles appear in the sun, light-coloured eyes;

– phototype III: reaction to the sun, sometimes gets sunburn, tans gradually. Fair skin, blond or light brown hair;

– phototype IV: reaction to the sun, rarely gets sunburn, tans easily. Light brown skin, light or dark brown hair, dark-coloured eyes;

– phototype V: reaction to the sun, rarely gets sunburn, tans easily. Brown skin, dark-coloured eyes;

– phototype VI: reaction to the sun, tans darkly, never gets sunburn. Black skin.

Pathophysiology

Defining the factors affecting pathophysiology is complex since they can also be intrinsic skin aging factors and risk factors for skin cancers.

UVB rays, lower-energy UVA and infrared rays that penetrate more deeply into the subcutis lead to oxidative stress with free radicals causing damage to DNA and cell membranes.

Both UVB and UVA rays are carcinogenic; it is UVA rays that classically bear greater responsibility for photoaging.

DNA damage can be seen resulting in a risk of skin cancers or an increase in p53 mutations.

Ultraviolet rays induce activation of AP1 pathways (activator protein 1), increasing the activity of MMP (matrix metalloproteinase), which degrades collagen and other components of the dermis.

Histology

There is thinning of the epidermis, cellular atypia, and increased melanogenesis.

Actinic elastosis is characterised by the accumulation of elastin in the superficial dermis causing the skin to appear yellowish.

The "Grenz zone" is a narrow subepidermal layer that demonstrates photoaging. This zone will increase during dermal remodelling with lasers or related technologies Fig. 3.

There is abnormal elastotic change, and fewer collagen fibres are present in the mid and deep dermis.

There are macromolecules such as proteoglycans and glycosaminoglycans in greater numbers, which present structural abnormalities and become deposited in the area of elastosis. They no longer fulfil their role of skin hydration, so the skin becomes dryer.

In proven photoaging, the vessels become less dense with thinner walls; the number of sweat glands falls and sebaceous glands are hyperplastic although secretion is not increased.

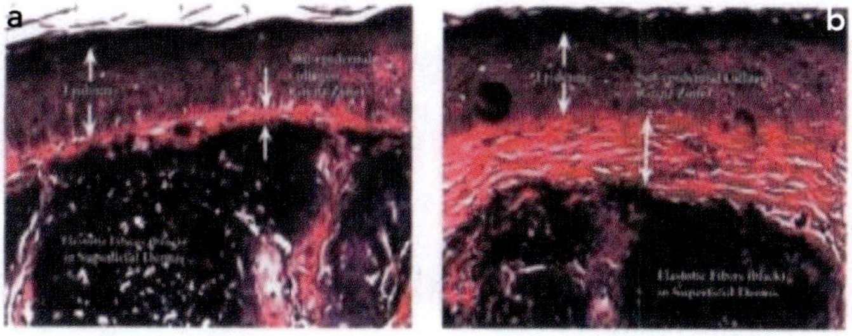

Figure 3 Histology after laser resurfacing

Biopsy before CO_2 laser resurfacing. The elastosis in the dermis is demonstrated by dark staining. Only a thin layer of normal collagen separates the epidermis from the dermis with elastosis (Fitzpatrick and Derstein 1996) (a)

Biopsy 12 weeks after CO_2 resurfacing. A significant increase in the Grenz zone can be seen with the presence of neocollagen (Fitzpatrick and Derstein 1996) (b)

Clinical features Fig. 4

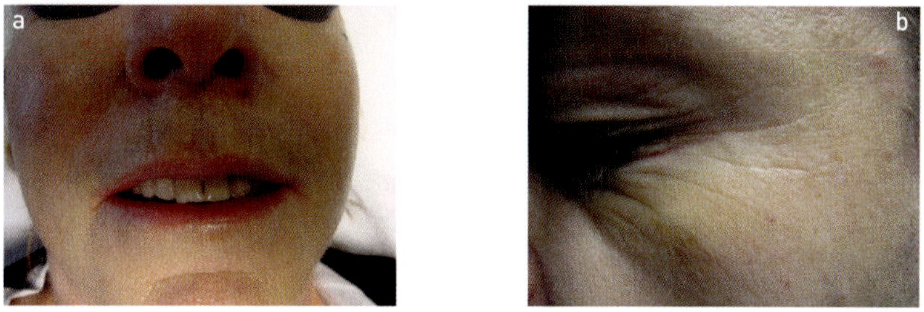

Figure 4 Perioral (a) and periorbital aging (b)

Dermatoheliosis

The lighter the phototype, and the more intense and prolonged the exposure to sunlight, the more marked photoaging will be in the areas exposed to the sun, which are the face, the lateral surfaces of the neck and the neckline.

On the face, the skin becomes dull or turns yellowish, presenting:

– actinic elastosis with dilated follicular orifices. The most extreme presentation is nodular elastosis with cysts and comedones (Favre-Racouchot syndrome); sebaceous hyperplasia around the highly seborrheic midline of the face;

– on exposure to UV rays, solar lentigines, actinic keratoses appear; telangiectasias;

– the skin gradually loses its elasticity, causing looseness;

– wrinkles appear in a perpendicular direction to muscle contraction: crows' feet, perioral and forehead wrinkles, frown lines, cheek wrinkles.

On the neck, the light-exposed areas of the lateral surfaces may show erythrosis interfollicularis colli, which can sometimes be pigmented, with a white area under the chin where the skin is protected from the sun by the chin.

On the back of the neck, thickened skin with deep wrinkles forming a criss-cross pattern.

Photocarcinogenesis

Photocarcinogenesis carries a risk of melanomas, basal or squamous cell carcinoma, and is often preceded by actinic keratosis, in particular on the nose, cheeks, or ears.

Glogau classification

This allows photoaging to be graded so that a suitable treatment for each type can be offered:

TYPE I (no wrinkles)

Patients under the age of 30
Mild pigment changes
Minimal wrinkles
Minimal or no make-up needed.

TYPE II (wrinkles in motion)

Age 30-40
Early visible solar lentigines (brown spots)
Keratosis palpable but not visible
Wrinkles on motion
Parallel smile lines beginning to appear
Foundation.

TYPE III (wrinkles at rest)

Over 50
Advanced photoaging
Discolouration, telangiectasias (red and pigmented stains)
Visible keratosis
Wrinkles even at rest
Heavy layer of foundation.

TYPE IV (only wrinkles)

Age 60-70
Yellowish-grey skin
Prior skin cancers
Wrinkles covering the skin
No longer use of foundation.

AGING OF THE SUBCUTANEOUS STRUCTURES

Over time, facial skin sagging, loss of subcutaneous fat volumes and bone resorption can be seen.

A young, rounded and plump face in the shape of a triangle with its base facing up gives way to a hollowed face with ptosis of the lower section, producing an inversion of the triangle shape with the base now at the bottom Fig. 5.

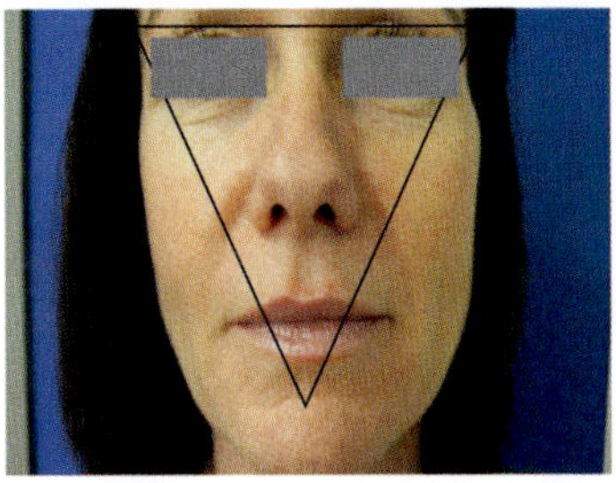

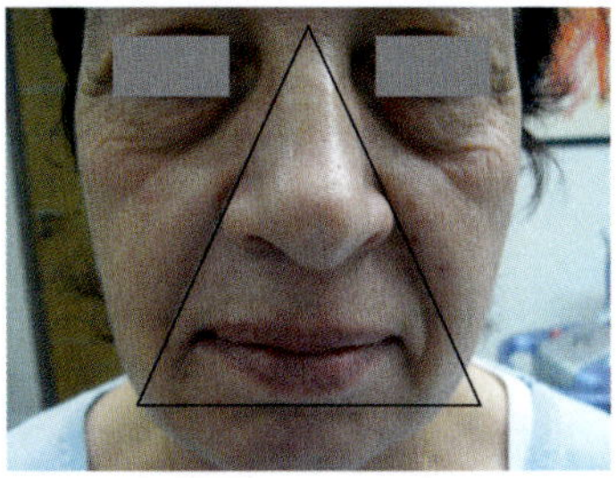

Figure 5 Ptosis and inversion of the triangle with aging

Ptosis of adipose tissue

The adipose tissue in the face sags and accumulates above the nasolabial folds, leading to a loss of cheek volume and increasingly bony appearance, and subsequently to ptosis of the lower cheek that changes the facial shape.

Thinning is often seen, with the facial appearance becoming bonier and the cheeks becoming hollower. Alternatively, the opposite can occur with the face becoming too full when there is an excess of adipose tissue causing ptosis and a double chin. The nasolabial folds grow longer to extend past the lips then becoming marionette lines Fig. 6.

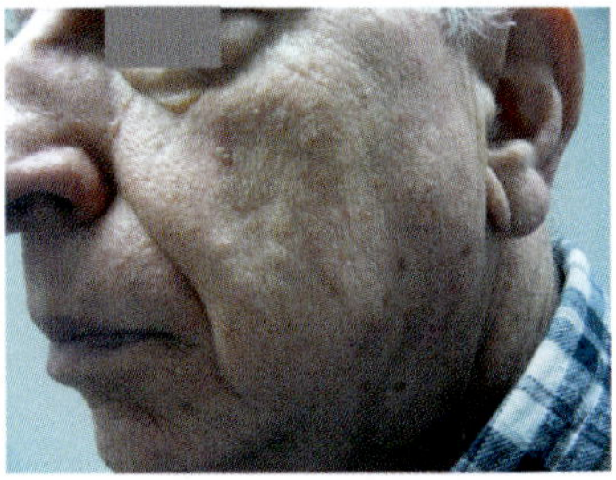

Figure 6 Accentuated nasolabial folds, lentigines, keratosis, sebaceous hyperplasia

Around the eye, hollowing or a pocket of fatty herniation below the lower eyelid can be seen with loosening of the upper eyelid and depression at the temples.

Some aging scales, in particular the Lemperle scale, suggest that aging should be graded focusing on zones Fig. 7 and 8.

Figure 7 Lemperle scale – Nasolabial fold

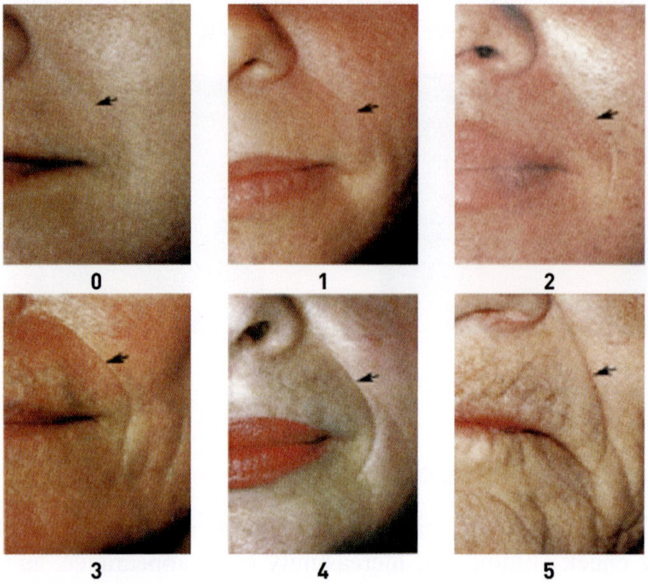

Figure 7 continued Upper lip wrinkles

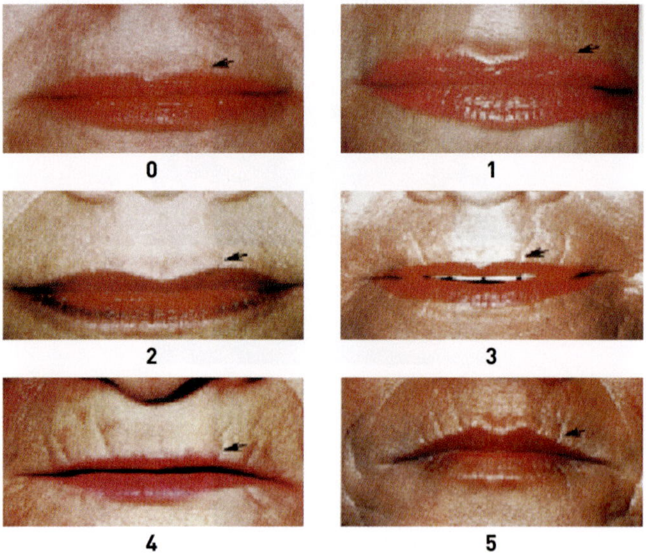

At each site the depth of the deepest wrinkle is evaluated, next to the arrows:

0 No wrinkles
1 Wrinkles barely visible
2 Superficial wrinkles
3 Moderately deep wrinkles
4 Deep wrinkles with well-defined edges
5 Very deep wrinkles/folds

Figure 8 Lemperle scale – Periorbital wrinkles

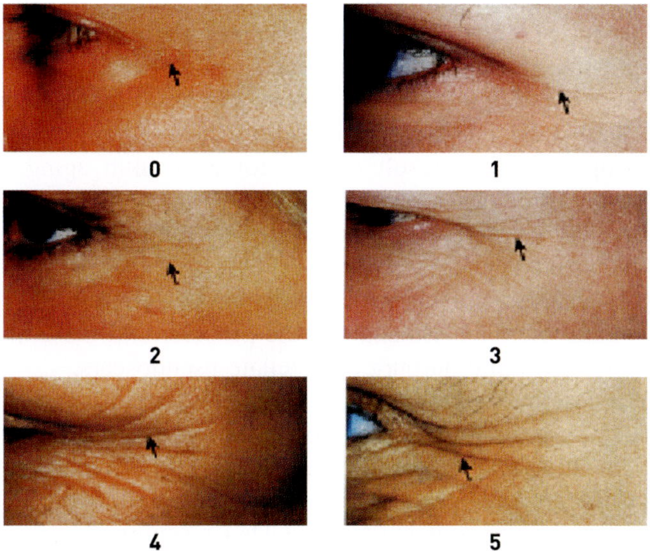

At each site the depth of the deepest wrinkle is evaluated, next to the arrows:

0 No wrinkles
1 Wrinkles barely visible
2 Superficial wrinkles
3 Moderately deep wrinkles
4 Deep wrinkles with well-defined edges
5 Very deep wrinkles/folds

Hypertonia and muscle fibrosis

Their signs can be seen in the upper part of the face with transverse forehead wrinkles, sagging eyelids, and more prominent frown lines.

In the lower part of the face, this muscular hypertonia accentuates marionette lines, sagging around the labial commissure, and chin lines.

In the neck, after transverse lines appear, atrophy and distension of the SMAS (superficial muscular aponeurotic system) lead to the platysma cords becoming visible.

Bone resorption

Bone resorption in the superior maxilla leads to a loss of supporting bone that accentuates perioral lines even further.

In the very elderly, this perioral bone resorption leads to collapse of the mouth structure, which in turn causes unattractive protrusion of the chin.

DERMATOPOROSIS

This term was suggested in 2004 by J.H. Saurat to be analogous with osteoporosis. It defines the state of extreme cutaneous fragility seen with aging across the whole integumentary system.

Dermatoporosis results from thinning of the dermis and epidermis and cutaneous atrophy that is clinically accompanied by gradual loss of skin viscosity and elasticity.

From around the age of 60, this "chronic cutaneous insufficiency syndrome" translates clinically into cutaneous atrophy with age-related purpura, pseudoscarring, and problems with wound healing. These manifestations can be observed more readily on the upper and lower limbs, the hands, and the neckline.

Primary dermatoporosis is a result of chronological skin aging and chronic sun exposure.

Secondary iatrogenic dermatoporosis is induced by long-term treatment with topical or systemic corticosteroids.

A number of clinical stages of dermatoporosis have been defined.

Stage I signs should alert the clinician to the process, and these are the significant thinning of the skin with senile purpura and stellate pseudoscars.

Stages II to IV are defined as stage I signs with additional lacerations and/or delayed wound healing that can progressively lead to the formation of dissecting haematomas. This latter stage constitutes a medical emergency and requires hospital admission. In terms of pathophysiology, dermatoporosis is related to a reduction in hyaluronic acid, in turn connected to a deficiency in cutaneous CD44 receptors that requires appropriate treatment.

CONCLUSION

A good understanding of facial skin aging allows for a thorough analysis of the patient's signs, both at rest and in motion, taking into account the different cutaneous and subcutaneous structures.

Classifications to define skin aging, zone by zone, have been put forward. In the future, a clear classification that takes into account signs both at rest and in motion would certainly lead to an improved consensus in terms of the treatments to offer.

Lasers and EBD lead to improved texture, reduced lines and wrinkles, better skin tone, and reductions in pigmented spots and telangiectasias.

Non-surgical management of skin aging is an overall approach that makes use of additional cosmetic treatments, skin peels, dermal fillers, and toxins.

Taking into account each patient's profile of skin aging and psychological outlook, a treatment plan will be offered that must preserve each individual face as far as possible and always have ethical concerns at the forefront. One should remember that the face cannot be treated without handling the neck, neckline, and hands, or addressing dermatoporosis affecting the whole integumentary system. As such, any treatment plan should be thorough and holistic.

REFERENCES

Beylot C. Vieillissement cutané: aspects cliniques, histologiques et physiopathologiques. Annales de dermatologie 2009; 136, sup 6: S263-S269.
Beylot C. Vieillissement cutané, prévenir-corriger-rajeunir. Edition med com 2007; 160.
Chung J, Cho S, Kang S. Why does the skin age? In Photo aging. Marcel Decker. Inc. 2004; 398.
Dahan S, Lagarde JM, Turlier V, Courrech L, Mordon S. Treatment of neck lines and forehead rhytids with a nonablative 1,540-nm Er:glass laser: a controlled clinical study combined with the measurement of the thickness and the mechanical properties of the skin. Dermatol Surg 2004; 30(6): 872-879.
Kaya G, Saurat JH. Dermatoporosis. A chronic cutaneous insufficiency/fragility syndrome: clinicopathological features, mechanisms, prevention and potential treatments. Dermatol 2007; 215: 284-294.
Saurat JH. Dermatoporosis; The Functional Side of Skin Aging. Dermatol 2007; 215: 271-272.
Turlier V, Rouquier A, Black D, Josse G, Auvergnat A, Briant A, Dahan S, *et al.* Assessment of the clinical efficacy of a hyaluronic acid-based deep wrinkle filler using new instrumental methods. J Cosm Laser Ther 2010; 12: 195-202.

CHAPTER 2

Basics of laser treatment

Paolo Bonan, Nicola Bruscino, Andrea Bassi,
Rossana Conti, Michela Troiano

LASER IN DERMATOLOGY: A CENTURY OF LASER

We are all surrounded by laser-based devices, but we usually exploit their functions without knowing it. Today, children are used to listening to music through MP3 players, while the previous generation used a laser system known as a "CD player"; probably very few people know much about the birth and development of lasers. The LASER device (Light Amplification by Stimulated Emission of Radiation) has numerous forebears. Einstein certainly made a great contribution to the creation of this kind of technology, and he is therefore considered as its "grandfather". He developed the theory about light travelling in waves of particles, photons, with the possibility of the stimulated emission of radiation, based on the previous concept introduced by Bohr, according to which the atoms emit energy moving from excited to resting statues [1]. The first precursor of the laser was the MASER (Microwave Amplification by Stimulated Emission of Radiation), launched in 1953 by several physicists. The interest in maser systems grew thanks to their use in radar technologies. Only in 1958 did Townes and Schawlow suggest that the maser concepts could be applied to optical and infrared regions. In the same year, Makow, Kikuchi, Lambe and Terhune generated a solid-state maser with numerous difficulties in finding an appropriate laser medium; they used crystalline corundum (ruby) in a large magnetic field. In 1959, Maiman continued exploiting the ruby maser, pumping ruby crystals through a special flash and producing red light at a wavelength of 694 nm. Following in 1961, several other masers, called lasers, were introduced: they were a great improvement due to the possibility of shortening the pulse duration to nanoseconds thanks to the Q-switching technology. The first dermatological applications were made by Goldman in 1961, the father of lasers in medicine. He used ruby laser for different dermatological conditions, publishing the effects on pigmented lesions such as hairs, tattoos, naevi as well as melanomas. He conducted promising studies on the treatment of vascular malformations with the argon laser, and on angiomas with the continuous neodymium:yttrium-aluminium-garnet (Nd:YAG) laser.

Only in 1964 was the continuous CO_2 laser invented, and then used for the photoexcision of tissues, like an optical scalpel; unfortunately the damage to the surrounding healthy areas, hypo/hyperpigmentation and scarring, limited the success of the early continuous wave lasers as ablative lasers, especially the argon laser [1]. In 1983, a revolutionary concept was introduced by Anderson and Parrish concerning selective photothermolysis, which has modified the way of exploiting laser properties; based on this concept, the operators can use lasers to selectively target and destroy the structures, while avoiding damage to the surrounding areas [2]. In the early 1980s, a new yellow-light dye laser was introduced for treating vascular lesions, through the absorption of light close to the absorption peaks of oxyhemoglobin. During the latter years of the 1980s, the Q-switched lasers (ruby, alexandrite and Nd:YAG) allowed dermatologists to achieve successful results for pigmented lesions as well as hair removal. In 1996 the erbium (Er):YAG laser with a typical wavelength of 2,940 nm became available on the market for superficial vaporization and possible skin resurfacing. The most recent advance in the long laser evolution was the fractional photothermolysis in 2003, which offered a huge variety of laser resurfacing procedures in dermatology [3].

The future that lies before us is very promising and bright: there is now a myriad of lasers and light-based devices for different dermatological lesions, all characterized by specific advantages and disadvantages, and offering a very favorable risk/benefit ratio, but only when performed by skilled dermatologists.

WHAT EXACTLY IS A LASER?

LASER (Light Amplification by Stimulated Emission of Radiation) is an optical resonator, consisting of two parallel reflective mirrors with an active solid (Nd:YAG, KTP, Er:YAG, Holmium:YAG, Alexandrite, Ruby, Titanium-sapphire laser), liquid (Pulsed Dye Laser) or gas (CO_2, Argon, Excimer, Helium-neon laser) medium between them. The active laser medium is a determining factor for the wavelength of the emitted photons. Moreover, the device needs a stimulation source of energy, called the pump portion of the system. The pumping part makes the laser medium extremely rich in atoms in excited state and poor in atoms in resting state. This condition, called the "population inversion", is crucial for the laser effectiveness. The pump can be a flash lamp, electrical current, or another pumping laser. The atoms of the laser medium, which are highly stimulated by the pumping part, move into an excited state and then emit their energy through the release of photons, which are repeatedly reflected between the two mirrors. However, since the exit mirror is only partially reflective, a part of these photons is emitted as a beam of light. The majority of lasers used in medicine, and mainly in dermatology, generate light in the ultraviolet (200-400 nm), visible (400-760 nm), near-infrared (760-1,400 nm), mid-infrared (1,400-3,000 nm), and infrared (> 3,000 nm) range. The typical features of laser light are monochromaticity, coherence and collimation; these characteristics differentiate laser light from non-laser light, such as Intense Pulsed Light (IPL). Laser light is monochromatic, being emitted with a clear and unique wavelength, coherent, since it consists of light waves in phase with the time and space, and collimated, as it does not diverge [4].

LASER-TISSUE INTERACTIONS

When the photons reach the surface of the skin, four different types of interaction may take place between the light and the skin: absorption, reflection, scattering, and transmission. In the majority of cases there is a combination of these interactions. The absorption of photons by a specific target in order to cause a biological effect is the scope of every laser treatment; during this process, all the energy delivered by the photons is transmitted to the target structures, the chromophores. Dermatological laser treatment changed radically in 1983 thanks to the introduction of the selective photothermolysis theory by Anderson and Parrish, defining how to localize thermal injury to the target tissue, thus minimizing the damage to surrounding areas by choosing the adequate wavelength of light that the chromophore inside the target tissue will absorb. The most important chromophores are hemoglobin, melanin and water, as well as porphyrins, flavin, retinol, nuclear acids, DNA, and RNA and external chromophores like tattoo ink. The absorption depends mainly on the matching of the wavelength of the photons with the absorption peak of a particular chromophore; light absorption by hemoglobin usually occurs at 415, 542, and 577 nm, while the absorption by melanin, ranging between 400 and 750 nm, is maximal in the ultraviolet area, decreasing throughout the visible region; in the near-infrared and the mid-infrared ranges, the tissue absorption is mainly due to water absorption. When the photons hit the skin surface, 4-6% of them are reflected by the tissue, which normally occurs in the stratum corneum of the skin, especially when dry or scaly. By increasing the angle of light incidence, we can induce a reflection that exceeds the 4-6% of the emitted photons. Reflection should be avoided since it causes a reduction in the fluence absorption by the target and therefore a loss of the laser effect. The photons may be scattered inside the skin, which mostly occurs with shorter wavelengths, especially in the superficial dermis, due to collagen fibers. The scattered photons lose the original direction of the incident light, creating irradiation to a larger area and thus losing a certain amount of energy. The photons, which have not been absorbed, reflected or scattered, undergo a transmission process via which they move to the deeper layers of the skin and subcutaneous tissues. Since the light penetration inside the skin is wavelength-dependent, the transmission only involves the photons with longer wavelengths, spared from scattering and able to reach deeper structures. The photons emitted by the Er:YAG laser (2,940 nm), at wavelengths near the water absorption peak, are not able to reach deep-seated structures despite the long wavelength, since the high water content in the superficial part of the skin induces intense absorption.

Light absorption in the skin can cause three different types of biological effects: photothermal, photomechanical, and photochemical. The most important for the success of the laser therapy is the photothermal effect (i.e. the energy of the irradiated photons is turned into heat due to the absorption of the photons by the chromophores). The effects may vary depending on the temperature reached in the target chromophore, the duration temperature elevation in the target, and the capacity of the target tissue to spread the heat to the surrounding tissues. With a temperature increase of 5° C one observes tissue injury and consequent inflammation; at 45-50° C there will be shrinkage of collagen fibers and reduction of enzymatic activity; at 60° C one can expect denaturation of proteins, membrane permeabilization, and coagulation of the collagen; at temperatures of 100° C there is formation of vacuoles, and higher than 100° C, tissue vaporization and carbonization; temperatures between 300 and 1,000° C result in thermoablation, photoablation and disruption of the tissue. The photomechanical effect occurs when very short laser pulses (nanoseconds or picoseconds) produce very strong energies: the tissue undergoes rapid thermal expansion, and an optical breakdown with intense shockwaves. This photomechanical effect is crucial for the Q-switched lasers that are able to disrupt the melanin and ink content of hyperpigmentation and tattoos, as well as being a determining factor for high-fluence, short-pulse, pulsed dye laser treatment of vascular disorders; the photomechanical damage, which clinically appears with purpura, is induced by short pulses and causes intravascular cavitation, vessel wall rupture, and hemorrhaging. The photochemical effect occurs when the absorbed photons affect the cellular metabolism or influence the signaling cascade. The consequences of the photochemical effect include increased cell proliferation and migration, modulation of growth factors, cytokines and other mediators, increased tissue oxygenation, and increased healing of wounds. Another example of the photochemical effect is evident with photodynamic therapy (PDT): an exogenous photosensitizer acts as a chromophore by absorbing light inside the target structure, and stimulating a selective photochemical reaction through the formation of singlet oxygen and radicals [5-6].

LASER DEVICES FOR THE DERMATOLOGIST

A large variety of different lasers and lights are currently used in the treatment of vascular lesions, even though more than one laser is often required to treat these lesions and achieve optimum cosmetic results:

Potassium Titanyl Phosphate (KTP) is a quasi-continuous laser which uses a neodymium:yttrium-aluminum-garnet crystal frequency-doubled with a KTP crystal to emit a 532-nm wavelength green light near the hemoglobin absorption peak. It is therefore useful in the treatment of superficial blood vessels. The main advantage of this kind of laser is the absence of post-op purpura, because it gradually heats the blood vessel without causing rupturing of the vessel wall or immediate purpura. It is mainly used for facial and leg telangectasias, but the shorter wavelength and low penetration depth restrict its use to superficial face, neck and chest lesions only. Due to its ability to match epidermal melanin absorption, it may be characterized by a higher risk of epidermal damage, especially in darker or tanned patients, thus limiting its use to Fitzpatrick skin types I-III [7].

Pulsed Dye Laser (PDL), which uses a rhodamine dye dissolved in a solvent and pumped by a flash lamp, emits a 585-600 nm wavelength yellow light, near the hemoglobin absorption peak. It is therefore considered the most specific laser currently available for the treatment of superficial vascular lesions. It was introduced in 1989 and used for telangectasias, hemangiomas, rosacea, although its best application is the Port Wine Stain (PWS) for which it is considered the treatment of choice with a high degree of efficacy and safety. It is also commonly used for treating Poikiloderma of Civatte. Despite its excellent efficacy and safety profile, the onset of purpura limits patients' acceptance as it may persist for 7-14 days after the laser session due to microvaporization of erythrocytes, vessel rupture and subsequent hemorrhage [8-20].

Alexandrite laser, which emits a 755 nm wavelength between the 532,595 nm and 1,064-nm lasers, belongs to the near-infrared category. At this particular wavelength the main chromophore is melanin, hence it is mainly used for hair removal and pigmented lesions; hemoglobin has a lower but significant absorption peak as well, so it can be used to treat deeper and resistant vascular lesions, such as reticular leg veins, mature and hypertrophic port wine stains, bulky vascular malformations, hemangiomas, and lymphangioma circumscriptum.

Diode lasers belong to the near-infrared range of lasers, emitting a wavelength between 800 and 980 nm. They target the third absorption peak of hemoglobin, and thanks to their longer wavelengths, penetrate deeper into tissues than lasers emitting in the green and yellow range (KTP and PDL). This enables their use for leg veins. The small spot size allows for treating smaller telangectasias, and since their wavelengths are poorly absorbed by melanin they can be used safely in skin types I-IV.

Neodymium:Ytrrium-Aluminum-Garnet (Nd:YAG) laser produces light in the infrared part of the spectrum at a wavelength of 1,064 nm. It is used for hair removal, but due to its low hemoglobin absorption peak and long wavelength it is also widely used for deep and resistant vascular lesions, PWS, and leg veins. Its increased penetration, as deep as 4-6 mm, may be painful for patients who often require anesthetics. The main advantage of the Nd:YAG laser compared to the other vascular lasers is the lower absorption coefficient by melanin, meaning that it can be used safely in darker skinned patients such as Fitzpatrick skin types IV-VI [21].

Erbium:Ytrrium-Aluminum-Garnet (Er:YAG) is a solid-state laser, characterized by the presence of erbium ions inside Ytrrium-Aluminum-Garnet or other crystals; it emits photons at wavelengths of 2,940 nm which are mainly absorbed by water in the superficial layers of the skin. This laser system is generally used for ablating the soft and hard tissues. It is a pulsed laser system with applications in dermatology, dentistry and invasive surgery. Its main drawback compared to other ablative lasers like CO_2 lasers, is its inability to induce coagulation. Er:YAG laser can be used with a fractional handpiece in a minimally ablative manner, especially for skin resurfacing.

CO_2 laser is a gas-state laser that emits photons at wavelengths of 10,600 nm. It offers a type of "No-Contact Surgery", since it enables accurate, efficacious and targeted thermal action on the lesions treated while protecting the surrounding tissues, thus guaranteeing optimal re-epithelization. This makes it suitable for surgical procedures since the limited inflammatory response is conducive to better healing. The extreme precision of the application means that the epidermis alone can be vaporized, or the thermal effect can be extended deeper into the papillary or reticular derma. The use of "color indicators" allows for step-by-step visual assessment of the depth reached and an accurate calculation of the clinical "end-point". This laser technique has also been used in the field of aesthetic medicine, exploiting its thermal rather than its vaporizing effects. Ablative resurfacing with CO_2 lasers has been considered the gold-standard for many years in the treatment of wrinkles, skin damage from photoaging and post-acne scars; however this method has also been associated with lengthy downtimes, occasional bacterial and viral infections, and bothersome side effects such as persistent erythema, post-inflammatory pigmentation alterations and possible atrophic scarring. The excellent results obtained with this technique have therefore stimulated research into methods and technologies capable of achieving similar results while reducing

downtimes and side effects. Based on these requirements, "fractional" resurfacing with CO_2 laser has been developped [22-30].

Fractional CO_2 laser is equipped with a scanning system, which makes it possible to obtain vertical micro-columns of damage, micro-ablative and micro-thermal zones (MAZs and MTZs), surrounded by areas of healthy tissue. Depending on the pulse used, the controlled release of heat in the treated micro-areas has an immediate tissue-shrinking effect and generates the stimulation of growth factors, wound repair, and the reorganization of new collagen. Another feature, which increases the versatility of this application is the possibility of selecting the distance (DOT spacing) between surrounding MAZs and MTZs, providing a resurfacing effect similar to the ablative technique with reduced spacing, or the more typical fractional effect, with greater spacing between DOTs. Each treatment session consists of numerous successive and consecutive pulses [1-5] in the same point without moving the scanner ("scalpel effect").

This function allows deeper penetration thanks to the possibility of repeating the laser emissions with the same parameters on one DOT before moving on to the next DOT during the same scanner passage Fig. 1 [31-40].

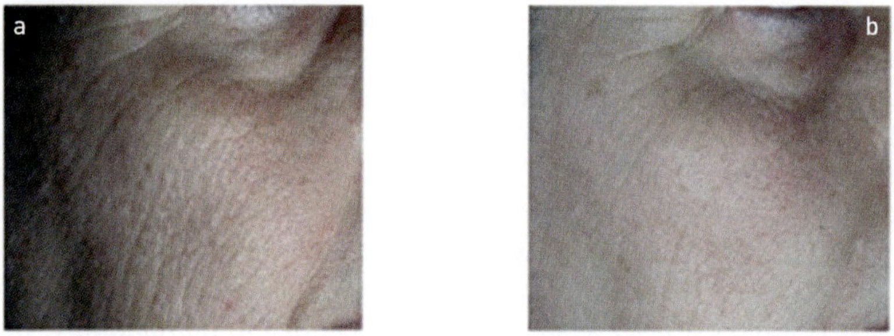

Figure 1 Before the treatments (a), excellent results after four sessions of fractional CO_2 laser (b)

New laser systems provide the right "pulse shape" and features for every single application the laser is engaged in. In these shapes the thermal tale can be varied dependently or independently of the energy content.

A laser company explored the possibility of applications of DOT therapy in sectors other than dermatology and aesthetic surgery. Thanks to its long experience in the production of CO_2 laser systems for gynaecology, the company developed a selective treatment called "MonaLisa Touch™": an innovative procedure for vulvo-vaginal atrophy, able to release energy through the special pulse while taking into account the peculiar features of the vaginal mucosa Fig. 2.

Fractional CO_2 laser combined with radiofrequency. For the last five years, bipolar radiofrequency devices have been considered non-invasive instruments, able to stimulate the deeper dermis in a non-ablative manner. Nowadays, some of these devices combine the effect of radiofrequency with laser or light energy in a unique tool capable of targeting aesthetical imperfections such as fine lines, wrinkles, pigment alterations, and skin laxity that have to be reduced or completely removed. These new laser systems simultaneously deliver fractional CO_2 laser and bipolar radiofrequency; the latter is able to amplify and enhance the effects of the CO_2 laser by remodeling the tissue in-depth,

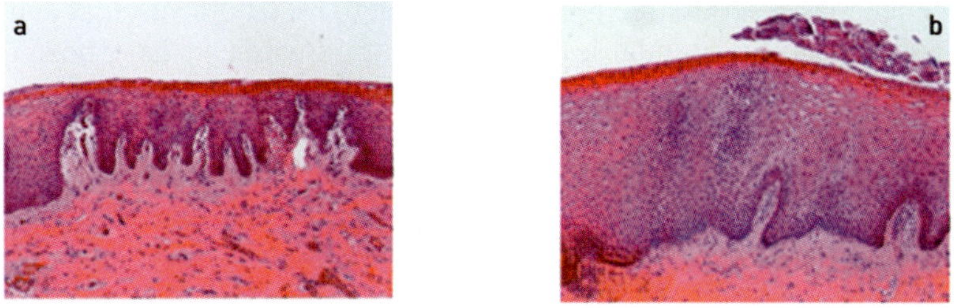

Figure 2 Vaginal mucosa under initial conditions. This morphology suggests vaginal atrophy which is at an early stage but that is also gradually evolving (a). Vaginal mucosa of the same patient a month after a treatment session with MonaLisa Touch. It is possible to see an increased number of epithelial layer (b)
(photos A. Calligaro, Professor of Istology and Embriology at University of Pavia-Italy)

toning flabbiness and stimulating fibroblast activity to produce new collagen. Previous histological studies have confirmed the presence of thickened, shortened collagen fibrils after bipolar radiofrequency treatments. An increased collagen-I up-regulation has also been observed.

The simultaneous emission of fractional CO_2 laser and radiofrequency yields several significant beneficial effects. In particular, there is a transfer of energy from the surface to the deeper layers with a more uniform lateral diffusion of the biostimulation. The laser-radiofrequency combination minimizes the amount of energy required from each system to achieve the desired results, decreasing the possibilities of side effects. Thanks to the combined use of laser and bipolar radiofrequency, skin tightening and rhytide reduction results can be achieved via the use of lower parameters, without the risk of side effects from higher settings **Fig. 3**. The average downtime for the fractional CO_2 laser/bipolar radiofrequency device is 5-6 days, which is a slight reduction compared to previous results using fractional CO_2 laser alone. A remarkable advantage is the control of erythema, both in terms of absolute intensity and duration. These aspects are vitally important for reducing the period of "social exclusion" imposed by the procedure [41-56].

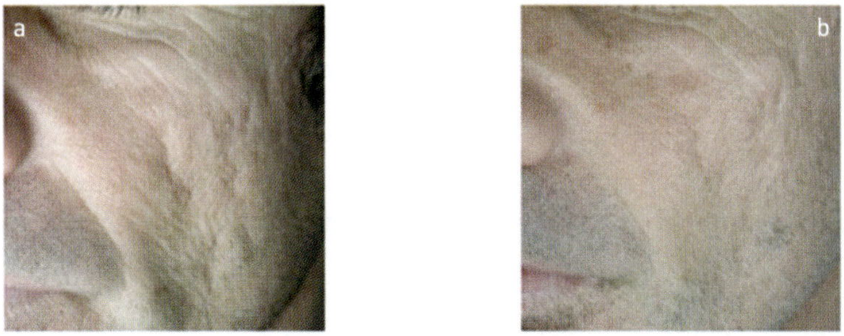

Figure 3 Before the treatments (a), a massive improvement of the wrinkles and the cutaneous texture after 4 sessions of fractional CO_2 laser combined with radiofrequency (b)

Intense Pulsed Light (IPL) emits polychromatic non-coherent broadband light in the 500-1,200 nm range, using cut-off filters to produce specific wavelengths capable of targeting vascular lesions more selectively. The advantage of this technique is its great versatility, which makes it possible for the physician to treat both vascular and pigmented lesions; regarding specific vascular lesions, successful treatments have been reported for PWS, hemangiomas, diffuse facial telangiectasias, and Poikiloderma of Civatte. One of the disadvantages of IPL is its bulky handpiece that makes maneuverability difficult, especially in anatomical parts like the small concave areas of the face, and its large dimensions; the use of a contact cooling gel also prevents real-time visibility of the area being treated [57].

HOW CAN A LASER BE USED?

Once the correct laser has been selected, the physician must decide on the most appropriate parameters, such as wavelength, spot size, fluence and pulse duration. The wavelength has to be chosen by considering the main chromophore inside the lesion, as well as its light absorption peak and depth. Q-switched laser at 532 nm is able to remove the superficial pigment of a brownish lentigo, whereas it can penetrate deep enough to remove black tattoo ink only if used at 1,064 nm. The spot size should match the diameter of the target structure as closely as possible to minimize damage to the surrounding tissues. The fluence can be considered the energy per unit area, and it is inversely proportional to the fraction of light absorbed by the target chromophore. Increased fluence must be used with chromophore-poor targets, deep skin targets and targets which barely absorb the wavelength. At the beginning of the first treatment session the dermatologist should choose the fluence according to the patient's pain threshold and in view of the clinical endpoint of that particular laser in use; in the majority of cases, the immediate response endpoint is given by the lesion clearance and the appearance of any typical side effects, such as mild purpura for the Pulse Dye Laser application. The last parameter to be selected is the pulse duration, which is determined by the thermal relaxation time (TRT) of the target, that is, the time the tissue takes to lose half the acquired heat which is proportional to the square of the target's diameter; the TRT of a larger structure will be longer than the TRT of a smaller structure. The pulse duration must be shorter than, or equal to, the TRT in order to limit the damage to the target tissue; if the duration is too short it could imply a loss of efficacy, whereas if the pulse is longer than the TRT the heat will spread to the surrounding structures, with the risk of possible scarring and other texture changes. In some cases the chromophore and the target are different, for example in the case of hair removal: the chromophore is the melanin contained inside the hair while the real target is the hair matrix, also containing melanin, and the hair stem cells inside the hair shaft, which do not contain it. In this case the heat diffusion required to destroy the surrounding structure is obtained with a longer TRT [58].

REFERENCES

[1] Bogdan Allemann I, Goldberg DJ (eds): Basics in dermatological laser applications. Curr Probl Dermatol Basel, Karger, 2011, vol. 42, pp. 1-6.
[2] Anderson RR, Parrish JA. Selective photothermolysis: precise microsurgery by selective absorption of pulsed radiation. Science 1983; 220: 524-527.
[3] Manstein D, Herron GS, Sink RK, Tanner H, Anderson RR. Fractional photothermolysis: a new concept for cutaneous remodeling using microscopic patterns of thermal injury. Lasers Surg Med 2004; 34(5): 426-438.
[4] Raulin C, Karsai S. Laser and IPL technology in dermatology and aesthetic medicine. Berlin, Springer-Verlag Heidelberg, 2011: 3-40.
[5] Watanabe S. Basics of laser application to dermatology. Arch Dermatol Res 2008; 300: s21-s30.
[6] Bogdan Allemann I, Goldberg DJ (eds): Basics in dermatological laser applications. Curr Probl Dermatol Basel, Karger, 2011, vol. 42, pp. 7-23.
[7] Kundu RV, Joshi SS, Suh KY, Boone SL, Huggins RH, Alam M, *et al.* Comparison of electrodessication and Potassium-Titanyl-Phosphate laser for treatment of dermatosis papulosa nigra. Dermatol Surg 2009; 35: 1079-1083.
[8] Karsai S, Roos S, Hammes S, *et al.* Pulsed dye laser: what's new in non-vascular lesions? JEADV 2007; 21: 877-890.
[9] Badawi A, Shokeir HA, Salem AM, *et al.* Treatment of genital warts in males by pulsed dye laser. J Cosmet Laser Ther 2006; 8: 92-95.
[10] Nowak KC, McCormack M, Koch RJ. The effect of superpulsed carbon dioxide laser energy on keloid and normal dermal fibroblast secretion of growth factors: a serum-free study. Plast Reconstr Surg 2000; 105: 2039-2048.
[11] Jimenez GP, Flores F, Berman B, *et al.* Treatment of striae rubra and striae alba with the 585-nm pulsed dye laser. Dermatol Surg 2003; 29: 362-365.
[12] Watson RE, Perry EJ, Humphries JD, *et al.* Fibrillin microfibrils are reduced in skin exhibiting Striae distensae. Br J Dermatol 1998; 138: 931-937.
[13] McDaniel DH, Ash K, Zukowski M. Treatment of stretch marks with 585 nm flashlamp pumped pulsed dye laser. Dermatol Surg 1996; 22: 332-337.
[14] Campolmi P, Brazzini B, Urso C, *et al.* Superpulsed CO_2 laser treatment of basal cell carcinoma with intraoperatory histopathologic and cytologic examination. Dermatol Surg 2002; 28: 909-912.
[15] Campolmi P, Troiano M, Bonan P, *et al.* Vascular based non conventional dye laser treatment for basal cell carcinoma. Dermatol Ther 2008; 21: 402-405.
[16] Tschachler E. Kaposi's Sarcoma. In: Fitzpatrick Dermatology in general medicine, 7th edn. U.S. McGraw-Hill, New York, 2007, pp. 83-1189.
[17] Schānermark MP, Raulin C. Treatment of xantelasma palpebrarum with the pulsed dye laser. Laser Surg Med 1996; 19: 336-339.
[18] Park HS, Kim JW, Jang SJ, *et al.* Pulsed dye laser therapy for pediatric warts. Pediatr dermatol 2007; 24: 177-181.
[19] Alster TS. Laser scar revision: comparison study of 585-nm pulsed dye laser with and without intra-lesional corticosteroids. Dermatol Surg 2003; 29: 25.
[20] Kuo YR, Wu WS, Jeng SF, *et al.* Activation of ERK and p38 kinase mediated keloid fibroblast apoptosis after flashlamp pulsed dye laser treatment. Laser Surg Med 2005; 36: 31-37.
[21] Schweiger ES, Kwasniak L, Aires DJ. Treatment of dermatosis papulosa nigra with a 1064 nm Nd:YAG laser: report of two cases. J Cosmet Laser Ther 2008; 10(2): 120-122.
[22] Riggs K, Keller M, Humphreys TR. Ablative laser resurfacing: high-energy pulsed carbon dioxide and erbium:yttrium-aluminum-garnet. Clin Dermatol 2007; 25: 462-473.
[23] Oni G, Mahaffey PJ. Treatment of recalcitrant warts with the carbon dioxide laser using an excision technique. J Cosmet Laser Ther 2011; 13: 231-236.
[24] Pozo J, Castineiras I, Fernandez-Jorge B. Variants of milia successfully treated with CO_2 laser vaporization. J Cosmet Laser Ther 2010; 12: 191-194.

[25] Madan V, Ferguson JE, August PJ. Carbon dioxide laser treatment of rhinophyma: a review of 124 patients. Br J Dermatol 2009; 161: 814-818.
[26] Boyce S, Alster TS. CO_2 laser treatment of epidermal nevi: long-term success. Dermatol Surg 2002; 28: 611-614.
[27] Cho SB, Kim HJ, Noh S, Lee SJ, Kim YK, Lee JH. Treatment of syringoma using an ablative 10,600-nm carbon dioxide fractional laser: a prospective analysis of 35 patients. Dermatol Surg 2011; 37: 433-438.
[28] Raulin C, Schoenermark MP, Werner S, Greve B. Xanthelasma palpebrarum: treatment with the ultra-pulsed CO_2 laser. Lasers Surg Med 1999; 24: 122-127.
[29] Aynaud O, Buffet M, Roman P, Plantier F, Dupin N. Study of persistence and recurrence rates in 106 patients with condyloma and intraepithelial neoplasia after CO_2 laser treatment. Eur J Dermatol 2008; 18: 153-158.
[30] Hunzeker CM, Weiss ET, Geronemus RG. Fractioned CO_2 laser resurfacing: our experience with more than 2,000 treatments. Aesthet Surg J 2009; 29: 317-322.
[31] Neaman KC, Baca ME, Piazza RC, VanderWoude DL, Renucci JD. Outcomes of fractional CO_2 laser application in aesthetic surgery: a retrospective review. Aesthet Surg J 2010; 30: 845-852.
[32] Karsai S, Czarnecka A, Junger M, Raulin C. Ablative fractional lasers (CO_2 and Er:YAG): a randomized controlled double-blind split-face trial of the treatment of peri-orbital rhytides. Lasers Surg Med 2010; 42: 160-167.
[33] Tierney EP, Hanke CW. Ablative fractionated CO_2 laser resurfacing for the neck: prospective study and review of the literature. J Drugs Dermatol 2009; 8: 723-731.
[34] Gotkin RH, Sarnoff DS, Cannarozzo G, Sadick NS, Alexiades-Armenakas M. Ablative skin resurfacing with a novel microablative CO_2 laser. J Drugs Dermatol 2009; 8: 138-144.
[35] Carniol PJ, Harirchian S, Kelly E. Fractional CO_2 laser resurfacing. Facial Plast Surg Clin North Am 2011; 19: 247-251.
[36] Ciocon DH, Engelman DE, Hussain M, Goldberg DJ. A split-face comparison of two ablative fractional carbon dioxide lasers for the treatment of photodamaged facial skin. Dermatol Surg 2011; 37: 784-790.
[37] Li YH, Chen JZ, Wei HC, Zhang L, Xu HH, Xu TH, Wu Y, Xu YY, Dong GH, Gao XH, Chen HD, Gold MH. A Chinese experience of fractional ultrapulsed CO_2 laser for skin rejuvenation. J Cosmet Laser Ther 2010; 12: 250-255.
[38] Chan NP, Ho SG, Yeung CK, Shek SY, Chan HH. Fractional ablative carbon dioxide laser resurfacing for skin rejuvenation and acne scars in Asians. Lasers Surg Med 2010; 42: 615-623.
[39] Omi T, Kawana S, Sato S, Bonan P, Naito Z. Fractional CO_2 laser for the treatment of acne scars. J Cosmet Dermatol 2011; 10: 294-300.
[40] Bonan P, Campolmi P, Cannarozzo G, Bruscino N, Bassi A, Betti S, Lotti T. Eyelid skin tightening: a novel "Niche" for fractional CO_2 rejuvenation. J Eur Acad Dermatol Venereol 2012; 26: 186-193.
[41] Newman J. Radiofrequency (GFX) ablation for the reduction of glabellar frowning. Facial Plast Surg 2010; 26: 266-273.
[42] Brightman L, Goldman MP, Taub AF. Subablative rejuvenation: experience with a new fractional radiofrequency system for skin rejuvenation and repair. J Drugs Dermatol 2009; 8: S9-S13.
[43] Paasch U, Bodendorf MO, Grunewald S, Simon JC. Skin rejuvenation by radiofrequency therapy: methods, effects, and risks. J Dtsch Dermatol Ges 2009; 7: 196-203.
[44] Montesi G, Calvieri S, Balzani A, Gold MH. Bipolar radiofrequency in the treatment of dermatologic imperfections: clinicopathological and immunohistochemical aspects. J Drugs Dermatol 2007; 6: 890-896.
[45] Sadick N. Bipolar radiofrequency for facial rejuvenation. Facial Plast Surg Clin North Am 2007; 15: 161-167.
[46] Geraghty LN, Biesman BS. Wrinkles and acne scars: technology-based treatment of periorbital wrinkles. In: Laser and IPL technology in dermatology and aesthetic medicine (Raulin C, Karsai S, eds) Springer-Verlag Berlin Heidelberg 2011; 299-305.
[47] Kim JE, Chang S, Won CH, Kim CH, Park KH, Choi JH, Lee MW. Combination treatment using bipolar radiofrequency-based intense pulsed light, infrared light and diode laser enhanced clinical effectiveness and histological dermal remodeling in Asian photoaged skin. Dermatol Surg 2012; 38: 68-76.
[48] Lee HS, Lee DH, Won CH, Chang HW, Kwon HH, Kim KH, Chung JH. Fractional rejuvenation using a novel bipolar radiofrequency system in Asian skin. Dermatol Surg 2011; 37: 1611-1619.

[49] Karsai S, Raulin C. Comparison of clinical outcome parameters, the Patient Benefit Index (PBI-k) and patient satisfaction after ablative fractional laser treatment of peri-orbital rhytides. Lasers Surg Med 2010; 42: 215-223.
[50] Tenna S, Cogliandro A, Piombino L, Filoni A, Persichetti P. Combined use of fractional CO_2 laser and radiofrequency waves to treat acne scars: a pilot study on 15 patients. J Cosmet Laser Ther 2012; Jun 1. In press.
[51] Prignano F, Bonciani D, Campolmi P, Cannarozzo G, Bonan P, Lotti T. A study of fractional CO_2 laser resurfacing: the best fluence through a clinical, histological, and ultrastructural evaluation. J Cosmet Dermatol 2011; 10: 210-216.
[52] Reilly MJ, Cohen M, Hokugo A, Keller GS. Molecular effects of fractional carbon dioxide laser resurfacing on photodamaged human skin. Arch Facial Plast Surg 2010; 12: 321-325.
[53] Trelles MA, Shohat M, Urdiales F. Safe and effective one-session fractional skin resurfacing using a carbon dioxide laser device in super-pulse mode: a clinical and histologic study. Aesthetic Plast Surg 2011; 35: 31-42.
[54] Sasaki GH, Travis HM, Tucker B. Fractional CO_2 laser resurfacing of photoaged facial and non-facial skin: histologic and clinical results and side effects. J Cosmet Laser Ther 2009; 11: 190-201.
[55] Prignano F, Campolmi P, Bonan P, Ricceri F, Cannarozzo G, Troiano M, Lotti T. Fractional CO_2 laser: a novel therapeutic device upon photobiomodulation of tissue remodelling and cytokine pathway of tissue repair. Dermatol Ther 2009; 22 Suppl 1: s8-s15.
[56] Saluja R, Khoury J, Detwiler SP, Goldman MP. Histologic and clinical response to varying density settings with a fractionally scanned carbon dioxide laser. J Drugs Dermatol 2009; 8: 17-20.
[57] Babilas P, Schreml S, Szeimes RM, Landthaler M. Intense Pulsed Light (IPL): a review. Lasers Surg Med 2010; 42: 93-104.
[58] Campolmi P, Bonan P, Cannarozzo G, Bassi A, Bruscino N, Arunachalam M, Troiano M, Lotti T, Moretti S. Highlights of thirty-year experience of CO_2 laser use at the Florence (Italy) department of dermatology. Scientific World Journal 2012; in press.

CHAPTER 3

Photorejuvenation of the face through laser treatment of vascular or pigmented lesions and LED

Anne Le Pillouer-Prost, Hugues Cartier

Differentiating between lasers to treat trophic changes connected to vasculature or pigmentation can be confusing in the context of photorejuvenation, because the clinical signs of dermatoheliosis or photoaging are often intermingled. The concept of the pigment, haemoglobin, and water absorption spectra is well known, and it governs which laser source will be best absorbed by the target, whether it be pigment, vasculature, or the intra- or extracellular aqueous medium.

FROM VASCULAR TO PIGMENTARY APPLICATIONS

It is not uncommon to find that patients who wish to reduce the appearance of broken capillaries through vascular laser treatment report an improvement not only in erythema but also in complexion, texture, and even dilated pores. Historically, vascular lasers were the first devices that demonstrated some efficacy in facial rejuvenation based on the concept of remodelling, which was popular in the 1990s.

The time has come to move on from the vascular laser because it is particularly common to see photodamaged skin that also presents vascular naevi, cherry haemangiomas, venous lakes, or rosacea.

The best-known lasers within the field of dermatology are 585 or 595 nm pulsed dye lasers [PDL] and the dual wavelength 1,064 nm long-pulsed Nd:YAG with 532 nm KTP, but copper vapour lasers should not be forgotten; admittedly they are less commonly used but they have very high photoselectivity for red chromophores. All of these lasers present strong affinity for oxy- and deoxyhaemoglobin apart from the 1,064 nm Nd:YAG, which is has an affinity for water and, to a lesser extent, methaemoglobin.

Most systems today have integrated cooling using air or cryogen spray, either continuously or on contact producing a "Peltier effect". This increases patient comfort but does not avoid post-operative developments.

If we consider the two best-known lasers (pulsed dye laser and 1,064 nm long-pulsed Nd:YAG), it has to be noted that while practitioners can offer either of these treatments for facial rejuvenation, they are diametrically opposed in terms of the ways in which they work and results they produce. Moreover, some systems like the Cynergy© Multiplex (Cynosure) now allow these two wavelengths to be used in a single pulse using 595 nm (not 585 nm) so that the absorption spectra of the different cutaneous targets are better covered, although this is at the expense of a precise and delicate calibration of the parameters.

The premise of rejuvenation based on the concept of laser remodelling ultimately rests on the stimulation of dermal fibroblasts, which receive their information from multiple cell-cell or cell-cytokine interactions. Two major routes can produce this stimulation: laser-induced vascular "shock" or heat "shock" responses lead to different activity markers being expressed, with variation over time (procollagen III production, expression at 3 months of αSMA, etc.). A laser-induced heat shock response will trigger changes in the profile of the renowned "heat shock proteins", which play a major role in modulating growth factors such as TGF-β, key elements in early inflammatory response and later cicatricial remodelling. However, if vascular laser injury is used to induce over-activation of blood components, especially platelets, this can equally trigger effects (release of powerful PDGF that stimulates fibroblasts, changes in the relationships of TGF-β subunits, etc.) that eventually lead to a dermal remodelling response. A best-case scenario would see certain lasers or their different configurations being combined to act on these two pathways to stimulation.

A PDL uses the principle of selective photothermolysis due to its wavelength and its mode of absorption. It is at once selective in terms of vasculature and it induces a relatively low temperature gradient in comparison with Nd:YAG. Thus, purpuric mode is a commonly used setting that often produces a startling outcome for the patient and their family but which rarely leads to serious consequences. When 1,064 nm Nd:YAG 1064 is combined with KTP 532 it becomes a laser that is effective both in the treatment of vascular disorders and superficial pigmented lesions but with such a strong affinity that it poses a risk of epidermolysis.

REJUVENATION AND PULSED DYE LASER

Fifteen years went by since Zelickson used a simple observational study to demonstrate a substantial reduction of moderate wrinkles in 20 patients after 12 months. This was achieved using 585 nm pulsed dye laser (spot size 6 mm, 0.45 ms, 3-6.5 J/cm^2), and yielded substantial reduction of moderate wrinkles of almost 50% for 9 patients out of 10 and up to 75% in 3 patients [1].

Numerous subsequent studies have produced contradictory or inconsistent results for both 585 nm and 595 nm PDL. Bjerring treated 40 patients with 585 nm PDL (spot size 4 mm, 0.45 ms, 2.4 J/cm^2) and showed pro-collagen production in areas that had undergone a single treatment, in contrast to areas treated a number of times, suggesting that there may not be a sound basis for claiming that a cumulative dose is needed for efficacy [2].

By contrast, Tanghetti saw only a modest impact on the reduction of eyelid wrinkles using multiple passes of the sub-purpuric mode of a 585 nm PDL [3].

Tay used a 595 nm PDL (spot size 10 mm, 10 ms, 7 J/cm^2, 40 ms spray before and 40 ms spray after, 30% overlap in a single pass) to treat the face in a small series of 10 patients (Glogau 1-2, phototype III-IV) over three sessions at two-month intervals. The results were graded as moderate by four patients with an improvement of less than 25%, five cases improved between 26 and 50%, and only one patient showed an improvement in excess of 50% between the treated and untreated halves of the face based on photographs before and after the sessions. The periorbital region pointed to some hope for better results than the cheeks or forehead. The authors reported only transient erythema and did not note any side effects [4].

In an observational study of 10 patients Bernstein used a 595 nm PDL but different parameters (spot size 10 mm diameter, 10 ms, fluence of 8-10 J/cm^2, delivered using the compression method on lentigines and ephelids) and showed that patients noticed a 72% reduction in facial vascular naevi and 65% reduction in hyperpigmentation, while 65% reported satisfaction in terms of reduced pores. There was even a 62% reduction in fine lines. Enthusiasm was more mixed from the observing doctors: 50% saw an improvement in fine lines, 82% in redness, 82% in vascular naevi, and 61.4% in pigmented lesions [5].

The problem lies with offering a vascular laser for rejuvenation only, with no major vascular target.

To put it clearly, it may be possible that the more vascular disorders there are to treat, the more rejuvenation will be induced as a result. This is highly possible based on a reading of individual experiences.

Vascular laser is perhaps not the most appropriate choice for erasing solar lentigines. It is possible to "cheat" by using a "compression" handpiece, however. This works by means of a translucent interface, supplied with some systems, using limited parameters that can be adapted for short pulses and high fluences (7 mm spot size, 1.5-3 ms, 9-16 J/cm^2), and foregoing the cooling system which is rendered ineffective by the compression interface. This was demonstrated by the Kauvar *et al.* study in 11 patients [6]. Purpura was almost non-existent for patients undergoing this compression treatment but the results were quite modest according to these authors and there were two cases of transient hypochromia.

We can therefore conclude that PDL is an unparalleled device in terms of safety. It is especially rare to see irreversible side effects reported when it is used for rejuvenation purposes. In terms of results, they are inconsistent and suitable indications are minor "vascular" dermatoheliosis with fine lines.

REJUVENATION AND LONG-PULSED 1,064 NM ND:YAG LASER

The long-pulsed 1,064 nm Nd:YAG laser is the "most blind" of vascular lasers. It carries its share of side effects, such as dermal necrosis if inappropriate settings are used or if the cooling method is ineffective.

In a dated publication, Lee reported an improvement of 10 to 30% after 3-6 treatments using 1,064 nm only, in 50 patients who underwent a single application (10 mm, 30-65 ms, 24-30 J/cm^2) [7]. Dayan *et al.* also reported a reduction in cutaneous laxity in 36% of 51 patients who were treated with a 1,064 nm device that was always used in isolation (10 mm, 22 J/cm^2, 50-ms) [8]. Some authors such as Douglas have furthermore demonstrated similar results in terms of laxity for both RF and Nd:YAG [9].

For the remodelling mode to be effective, it must entail a conversion of photons into a raw source of heat or it must set off the previously described cascade of pathophysiogenesis gradually over a longer period. The parameters used in previous studies, with long pulse durations and high fluences induce a very sudden and noticeable rise in tissue temperature with almost no side effects, apart from the rather intense pain that serves as an "endpoint" in practice. This "pricking" pain that demonstrates the thermal injury must remain brief and transform into a simple sensation of warmth with the treated area showing visible erythema immediately and lasting for a few hours. Some practitioners therefore suggest prioritising alternative settings in order to achieve the same goal while allowing for greater tolerability during the sessions. Such alternative settings include using a large spot size (8-10 mm), much lower fluences (5-10 J/cm^2), and very brief pulses (0.5-3 ms) with multiple pulse-stacked sweeps over the area using a beam that is defocused 3-4 cm away. The end-point is the mild but prolonged erythema obtained after 3,000-6,000 pulses, depending on the area treated. The best approach is to use temperature sensors in order to be sure that the external cutaneous temperature is stabilised at over 40° C (with a maximum of 47° C) for several minutes.

Mild oedema of the treated area may be reported. The sessions are entirely pain-free and need to be repeated using the same method as before, with an average of four to six treatments at three or four-week intervals, in order to see a change in texture with a reduction in erythrosis and a return to firm skin. Using this method of gradual collagen stimulation, all phototypes, from I to VI, can be treated.

REJUVENATION AND 532 NM KTP LASER

Its short wavelength makes this type of laser particularly effective in the treatment of erythrosis and broken capillaries, which are usually vascular naevi. The latest systems combine a large spot size and the Peltier effect at 5° C for cooling, which renders the older scanning systems that compensate for the smaller spot size of their pulses obsolete. The usual settings are between 5 and 10 J/cm^2 and the pulse duration is between 5 and 15 ms for spots sizes of 3-12 mm^2. It is important to consult the graphs for each system and to run a test that triggers immediate disappearance of vascular naevi and lentigines to turn greyish, however.

KTP laser is also effective for the removal of even the lightest solar lentigines, as long as the patient's phototype is below IV or even III, to be on the safe side. When used for rejuvenation, experience must prevail in order to avoid a reticular pattern or on the contrary pulse stacking in one area, which can be a source of epidermolysis, but ultimately the 532 nm KTP laser restores brightness to skin that has become dull.

Usually this is followed by oedema or redness lasting from a few hours to a few days with small crusts; these signs correspond to the destruction of solar lentigines [10].

It is sensible to combine this with long-pulsed Nd:YAG because this adds the absorption by the three major cutaneous targets needed for thermal injury to an undeniable action on the complexion.

REJUVENATION WITH 578 NM YELLOW LASER AND 511 NM COPPER VAPOUR LASER

This device is rarely used but, because of its wavelength, it is particularly effective in the destruction of vessels and lentigines [11].

REJUVENATION WITH LONG-PULSED ALEXANDRITE LASER

Equally, long-pulsed alexandrite lasers, usually used for hair removal, can quite selectively destroy epidermal pigmented lesions when applied using several successive pulses with appropriate settings (small spot sizes of around 5 mm for fluences of 20-25 J/cm^2 and pulse durations of 5 ms). Lentigines take on a greyish or blackish appearance and then flake off within a few days. In order to combine thermal remodelling with a brightening of the area to be treated, successive pulses can be stacked for lentigines and then the whole area can be treated with the laser beam. In that case, care must be exercised to use wide diameter spots, from 10 to 18 mm, lower fluences of around 15 to 20 J/cm^2 and pulse durations of 25 to 50 ms. It is also important to take care in hairy areas that absorb photons.

REJUVENATION AND TREATMENT OF PIGMENTED LESIONS USING Q-SWITCHED LASER: THE GOLD STANDARD

In the management of facial rejuvenation, it is crucial to take into account the brightness of the complexion and any solar lentigines that pepper the skin surface. The initial consultation should clearly lead to the exclusion of patients who present dyskeratosis with any extent of pigmentation, carcinomas, and lentigo maligna melanomas, which are differential diagnoses of lentigines.

The gold standard lasers are those that emit pulses in a few nanoseconds, known as Q-switched lasers and including the 594 nm ruby laser, 532 nm KTP laser, and 755 nm alexandrite laser. They have the ability to be both photoselective because of their high affinity for the pigment and photoacoustic due to a phenomenal level of energy being delivered in a very short space of time. The treatments are very quick because of pulse emission of up to 10 impacts/second for spot sizes of 2-6 mm. This means that the emission duration is very short so the sensation of heat is bearable and due to their high affinity for the pigment, they combine selectivity with efficacy. The practitioner can choose to treat lentigines only, but using varied fluence parameters it is wise to treat the whole anatomical area in order to achieve an even appearance. The results are striking, tailored to need, and can be achieved in one or several sessions, with a comparable aftermath to that seen with a medium-depth skin peel, consisting of desquamation and small crusts that flake away within a few days, leaving behind clear and glowing skin. Naturally, these lasers are principally for use in phototypes I to III because in any higher phototype, the risk of post-inflammatory pigmentation is greater in more than 1/3 of cases, or there may even be major and sometimes permanent hypochromia.

At 532, 694 and 755 nm, rejuvenation of the complexion is addressed above all, through the destruction of lentigines. Each impact results in flocculation in the epidermis through vacuolisation of the keratinocytes with whitening of the skin in the same way as with tattoo removal. The more intense the snowy white appearance, the more the effect of a skin peel is achieved, with crusts of varying intensity and a lengthy healing process Fig. 1-3.

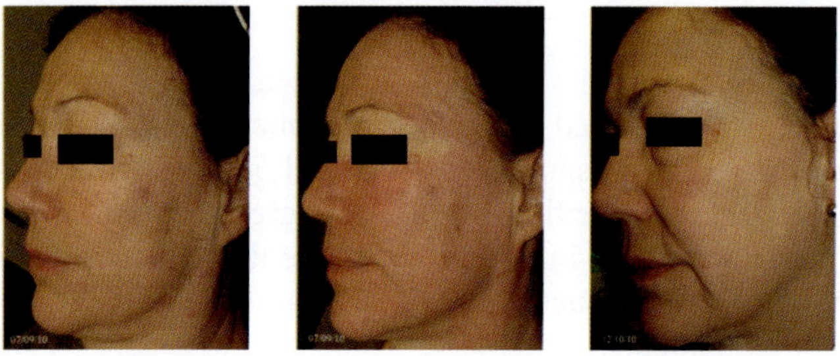

1 2 3

Figure 1, 2, 3

1 Before Q-S 532 nm laser treatment
2 Laser-peel mode 0.8 J/cm^2 diameter 6 mm sweeping over the whole face 3 times following lentigine-focused pulses of 4 J/cm^2 diameter 4 mm
3 Very clear improvement with photorejuvenation 5 weeks after a single 532 nm QS laser-peel session

Friedman had already reported on the value of using the 1,064 nm Q-switched laser in 2002 after analysis using biomechanical and photographic three-dimensional images. In three to five sessions, his team noted transformation of cutaneous texture in terms of smoothness, reduced rough patches, lines and scars, both for sun-damaged and acne-scarred skin [12]. In 2008, Liu published a comparative histology study looking at 595 nm pulsed dye laser, 1,064 nm Nd:YAG, 1,320 nm fractionated laser, and 1,064 nm Q-switched Nd:YAG laser. The Q-switched laser increased fibroblast levels by nearly 60%, as opposed to 30-35% for the other modalities, triggering the production of hydroxyproline, a marker of collagen production. More importantly, it was the only modality to trigger the reappearance of the "essential" collagen type III that is only seen during foetal development and in childhood, in addition to collagen type I production [13].

Ultimately, Q-switched lasers, previously confined to tattoo removal, have turned out to be the gold standard when compared to other photon devices.

In terms of settings for 1,064 nm mode, we look for the pinpoint petechiae that point to injury to the dermis and vessels. However, by increasing fluences or using dual-pulsed or quasi long-pulsed modes exceeding 200 ns, the thermal effect is increased leading to proven remodelling. By contrast, the photomechanical effect can be prioritised by transforming the new generation Q-switched lasers that use a "flat top" or "top hat" beam distribution into a form of Gaussian beam. The pulse is defocused more than 10-15 cm away from the skin while spot size is artificially reduced by adjusting the directional control on the handpiece without changing the recommended system parameters for photoremodelling; this means that the light beam is concentrated for a greater photoacoustic effect. For example: for a 1,064 nm laser, a spot diameter calibrated at 6 mm, and a fluence of 8 J/cm^2, the spot size of the handpiece could readily be reduced to 4 mm or even 3 mm, at a distance of 10-15 cm from the skin, with the goal of treating deep wrinkles. Intense purpura results, or even suffusion haemorrhage that can sometimes be striking resulting from involvement of at least the papillary dermis and its source capillary network. This action is at once mechanical and vascular and it induces a process of tissue repair and collagen stimulation. This technique remains to be validated by the manufacturers and requires training Fig. 4-6.

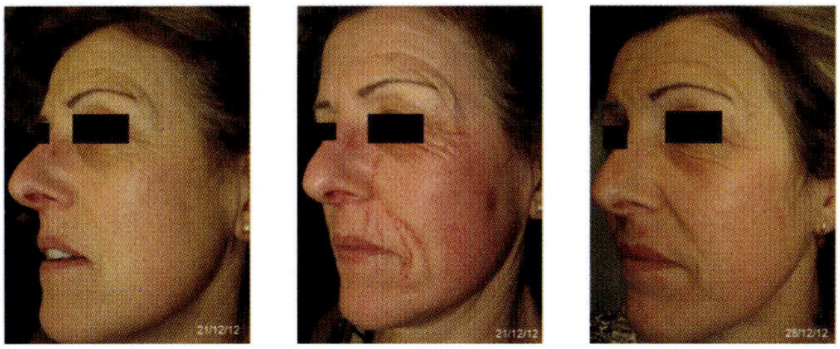

4 5 6

Figure 4, 5, 6

4 Before photon remodelling with 1,064 nm Q-switched laser
5 Dual-pulsed wrinkle treatment mode 5.6 J/cm^2; diameter 6 mm; swept over the face to achieve petechiae and focused on the wrinkles using single-pulsed mode 8 J/cm^2 with multiple passes, spot diameter 4 mm but defocused 10 cm away for better collagen induction with dermal vascular injury
6 Result after one session and healing in less than 8 days after reduction of fine lines

At 1,064 nm, Q-switched laser is active on dermal pigmentations but this means it is becoming an increasingly serious contender in photon remodelling to rival non-ablative lasers. The combination of at least two of these wavelengths in one session, usually 532 nm and 1,064 nm, means that both the dermis and the epidermis can be treated at the same time, i.e. the dermal collagen structure and the complexion.

LED

The use of LEDs to manage vascular and pigmented lesions is a source of some debate. There is a major paradox in the literature regarding in vitro work in which the majority of authors have published convincing results for inflammation, healing, clearing lentigines, and brightening complexion. Yet the clinical results clash with these. Among the first publications were those from Weiss and McDaniel [14]. They reported on a series of 93 patients who were treated with an LED system emitting a spectral band of 590 nm, placed 2 cm away from the face (pulsed, 0.15 J/cm^2, less than 1 minute of exposure) during eight sessions spread over four weeks: there was an improvement in periorbital wrinkles in 56% of subjects, in skin texture for 87%, in erythema in 65%, and in pigmentation in 62%. In a double-blind study in which 53 subjects were treated with 660 nm red LED, Barolet *et al.* [15] reported mean improvement in fine lines of 24.6 µm and, in one case, 225.5 µm. Similarly, other authors such as Russell [16] and Lee [17] have demonstrated the value of combining dual spectral bands consisting of red and infrared (830 nm) with results that were interesting both in terms of clinical improvement, and in terms of histology or immuno-histochemical profiling.

However, Boulos *et al.* [18] in 2009 were not alone in reporting an absence of effect on rejuvenation with a 590 nm LED system in a study that made quite a sensation in the community using LEDs. This means that for pure rejuvenation, we are able to cite the earliest publications only, dating from almost a decade ago, using spectra between 590 nm and infrared for exposures of a few minutes with results on the complexion and lines. Conversely, the most recent publications have put forward only very modest results. Just as the complementary nature of LEDs and 5-ALA or MAL in the context of photodynamic therapy is interesting in terms of results while not always being flexible in terms of expected effects, there is a need for effective and reproducible protocols in the usage of LEDs only that include the light sources available today to be better defined and evaluated.

CONCLUSION

All of these photon devices are useful for photorejuvenation. Each one has individual physical characteristics due to its wavelength and method of photothermal, photoselective or photomechanical emission, but they all produce changes to skin texture and complexion that are ultimately relatively similar. It is up to the practitioner to choose the device that is most appropriate for fulfilling the patient's request.

REFERENCES

[1] Zelickson BD, Kilmer SL, Bernstein E, *et al.* Pulsed dye laser for sun damaged skin. Lasers Surg Med 1999; 25: 229-236.
[2] Bjerring P, Clement M, Heickendorff L, Egevist H, Kiernan M. Selective non-ablative wrinkle reduction by laser. J Cutan Laser Ther 2000; 2: 9-15.
[3] Tanghetti EA, Sherr EA, Alvarado SL. Multipass treatment of photodamage using the pulse dye laser. Dermatol Surg 2003; 29: 686-690.
[4] Tay YK, Khoo BP, Tan E, Kwok C. Long pulsed dye laser treatment of facial wrinkles. J Cosmet Laser Ther 2004; 6(3): 131-5.
[5] Eric F. Bernstein, The New-Generation, High-Energy, 595-nm, Long Pulse-Duration Pulsed-Dye Laser Improves the Appearance of Photodamaged Skin Lasers in Surgery and Medicine 2007; 39: 157-163.
[6] Kauvar AN, Rosen N, Khrom T. A newly modified 595-nm pulsed dye laser with compression handpiece for the treatment of photodamaged skin. Lasers Surg Med 2006; 38(9): 808-813.
[7] Lee MW. Combination 532-nm and 1,064-nm lasers for noninvasive skin rejuvenation and toning. Arch Dermatol 2003; 139: 1265-1276. Erratum In: Arch Dermatol 2004; 140: 1265.
[8] Dayan SH, Vartanian AJ, Menaker G, Mobley SR, Dayan AN. Nonablative laser resurfacing using the longpulse (1,064-nm) laser. Arch Facial Plast Surg 2003; 5: 310-315.
[9] Douglas JK. Single-treatment skin tightening by radiofrequency and long-pulsed, 1,064-nm Nd: YAG Laser compared. Lasers Surg Med 2007; 39: 169-175.
[10] Butler EG, McClellan SD, Ross EV. Split treatment of photodamaged skin with KTP 532 nmLaser with 10 mm handpiece versus IPL:A cheek-to-cheek comparison. Lasers Surg Med 2006; 38: 124-128.
[11] Owen WR, Hoppe E. Copper bromide laser for facial telangiectasia: a dose response evaluation. Australas J Dermatol 2012; 53(4): 281-284.
[12] Friedman PM, Skover GR, Payonk G, Kauvar AN, Geronemus RG. 3D in-vivo optical skin imaging for topographical quantitative assessment of non-ablative laser technology. Dermatol Surg 2002; 28(3): 199-204.
[13] Liu H, Dang Y, Wang Z, Chai X, Ren Q. Laser induced collagen remodeling: a comparative study in vivo on mouse model. Lasers Surg Med 2008; 40(1): 13-19.
[14] Weiss RA, Weiss MA, Geronemus RG, McDaniel DH. A novel non-thermal non-ablative full panel LED photomodulation device for reversal of photoaging: digital microscopic and clinical results in various skin types. J Drugs Dermatol 2004; 3(6): 605-610.
[15] Barolet D. In vivo human dermal collagen production following LED-based therapy: the importance of treatment parameters. Lasers Surg Med 2005; Supp 17: 76.
[16] Russell BA, Kellett N, Reilly LR. A study to determine the efficacy of combination LED light therapy (633 nm and 830 nm) in facial skin rejuvenation. J Cosmet Laser Ther 2005; 7(3-4): 196-200.
[17] Lee SY, Park KH, Choi JW, Kwon JK, Lee DR, Shin MS, Lee JS, You CE, Park MY. A prospective, randomized, placebo-controlled, double-blinded, and split-face clinical study on LED phototherapy for skin rejuvenation: clinical, profilometric, histologic, ultrastructural, and biochemical evaluations and comparison of three different treatment settings. J Photochem Photobiol B 2007 27; 88(1): 51-67.
[18] Boulos PR, Kelley JM, Falcão MF, Tremblay JF, Davis RB, Hatton MP, Rubin PA. In the eye of the beholder – skin rejuvenation using a light-emitting diode photomodulation device. Dermatol Surg 2009; 35(2): 229-239.

CHAPTER 4

Facial skin aging and Intense Pulsed Light (IPL)

Catherine Raimbault

Intense Pulsed Light (IPL), or flashlamp therapy, was invented 20 years ago by Dr Eckhouse, who demonstrated that a light source and appropriate filters could be used for a variety of applications and for the treatment of noticeably larger areas than lasers. His theory was based on the performance of lasers that had already been used for medical purposes for many years. The operating principles of intense pulsed light systems are identical to those of thermal lasers: the light energy delivered by the device is transformed into heat when absorbed by a chromophore and that heat (approximately 65° C) destroys the targeted structure. However, chromophores all have specific characteristics: each has its own light absorption peaks limited to narrow absorption spectrum. Therefore, a given chromophore may have absorption peaks at different wavelengths and consequently react to light of different colours.

WHAT IS INTENSE PULSED LIGHT AND HOW DOES IT DIFFER FROM LASERS?

Intense pulsed light systems are typically made up of the following:

- a casing containing an energy generator, a light source, a computer control module, a cooling system;
- a handpiece (or applicator) including a flashlamp containing xenon in most cases, a reflector enabling the redirection of a maximum of photons and therefore light towards the skin, a filter which blocks out certain wavelengths, a light guide that is placed in contact with the skin via a quartz or sapphire block, which is essential when the handpiece has a skin contact cooling system.

Unlike laser therapy which diffuses small-diameter monochromatic rays in perfectly parallel and coherent light beams, intense pulsed light devices use defocused Tab. 1 and non-coherent broad spectrum polychromatic light (from 300 nm to 1,200 nm and

Table 1

Intense pulsed light	Laser
Polychromatic (range of wavelengths)	Monochromatic (only one wavelength)
Non-coherent (the photons are not in-phase)	Coherent (the photons are always in-phase)
The light is defocused	The light beams are parallel (directional light)

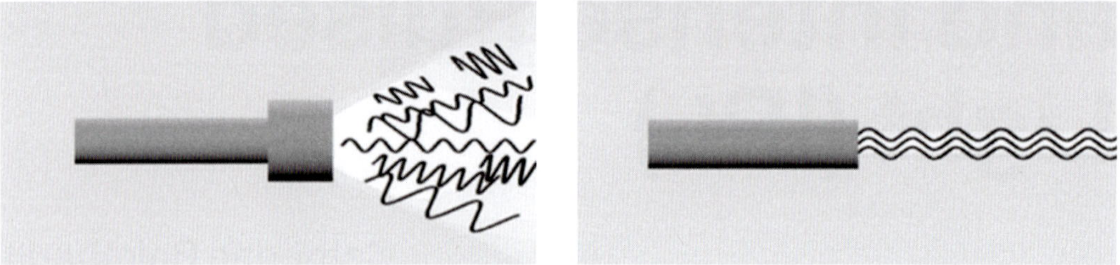

sometimes even 1,400 nm) in the ultraviolet light, visible light (violet to red) and near-infrared ranges.

The advantages of pulsed light are immediately obvious: filters can be used to narrow the spectrum of pulsed light to obtain wavelengths that act on selected chromophores whereas laser light, consisting of only one wavelength and consequently just one colour, can be used to target only one chromophore. Over the years, manufacturers have produced a wide selection of filters for a maximum of applications and the wavelengths for a given indication (hair removal, treatment of vascular or pigmented lesions, acne, photo-rejuvenation, etc.) can vary significantly depending on the brand of the devices. Each manufacturer proposes a "unique" solution based on several parameters combined with the choice of wavelength, i.e. the number of pulses, their duration, the search for the best compromise between absorption and depth of penetration. However, ultraviolet light, i.e. with a wavelength shorter than 400 nm, which is particularly dangerous for the skin and eyes, is blocked out in all cases. In 1997, the technology was considered to have been significantly improved when a Danish company presented a new generation of intense pulsed light devices. The technology employs dual-mode filtering of the wavelengths as illustrated in Fig. 1. In addition to filtering out the light with shorter wavelengths (through different coloured glass plates) leaving only those required for a given treatment, the system also filters out all the wavelengths above 950 nm using the water from the cooling system and a patented technique.

Dual-mode filtering has two advantages, i.e. it improves treatment efficacy and safety. Above 950 nm, the only chromophore left in the skin is water. In other words, a non-negligible portion of thermal energy is wasted on an ineffective chromophore and, if treatment of the target chromophore (melanin or haemoglobin) is to be effective, fluence needs to be increased substantially, which increases the risks and the discomfort for the patient. Subsequently, another company used the same principle and a slightly different technology to divide the spectral range into two groups of wavelengths with a filtered zone in-between. Another feature that is important for the efficacy and safety of intense pulsed light devices is pulse shape. With numerous devices, the pulse is delivered with increasing intensity to peak fluence before decreasing progressively, in the style of a light dimmer. This presents two drawbacks: firstly, the spectral range is not homogeneous

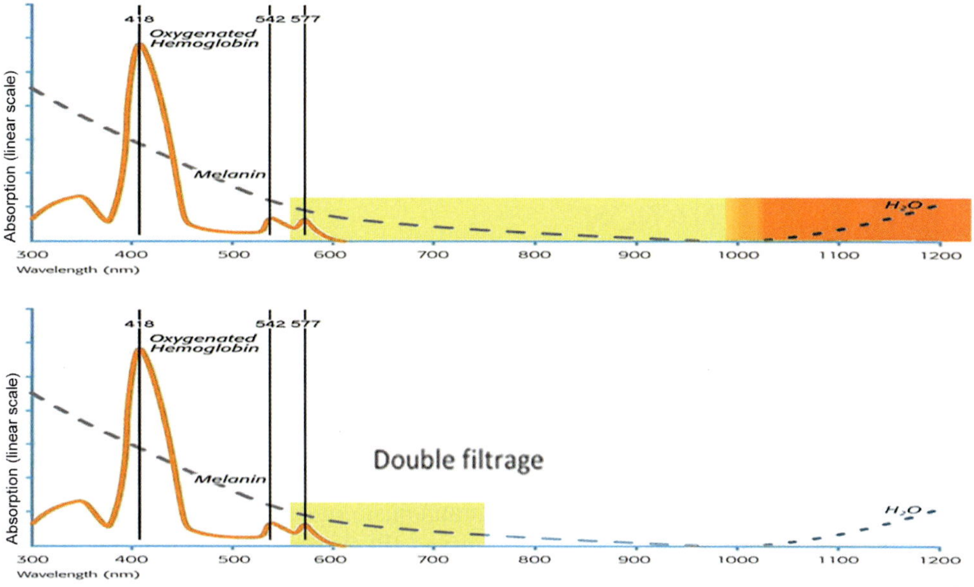

Figure 1 Dual-mode filtering of the wavelengths

during the pulse; secondly, to compensate the lesser energy in the ascending and descending phases and therefore to preserve the set fluence throughout the duration of the pulse, peak fluence must be significantly higher than the set value. This translates into an increase in risk and discomfort. It is therefore generally admitted that the ideal pulse is obtained with what is referred to as square pulse technology, which uses a complex start/stop mechanism allowing an almost instantaneous rise in intensity and a stop just as sudden. Figure 2 shows the two different pulse shapes.

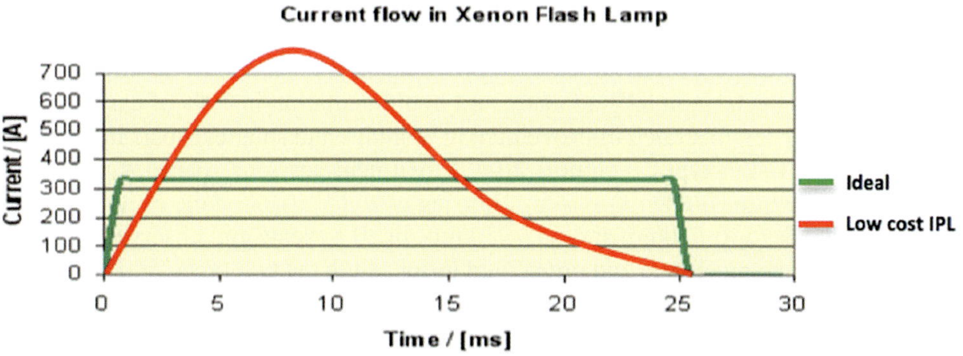

Figure 2 Two different pulse shapes

The other points to be considered in a pulsed light device are the ergonomics of the handpiece (weight, size of the luminous spot, visibility of the treatment), the lifespan of the lamps and the cost of their replacement or their reconditioning. The computer program is also essential: does it have pre-programmed settings, what are the possibilities for tailoring treatment to individual needs for experienced operators, what is the range of pulse durations, are they determined as a function of the various possible sizes of the target, a decisive parameter for the success of numerous treatments?

INTENSE PULSED LIGHT FOR FACIAL SKIN PHOTOREJUVENATION

Intense pulsed light when used for facial skin photorejuvenation exerts an effect at three different levels: it acts on vascular lesions (erythrosis, telangiectasia), pigmentation and skin texture.

Clinical studies

Since the 2000s, many histological or immunohistological studies have tried to describe the tissue modifications observed following IPL treatment: collagen remodelling, reduction of solar elastosis [20], increase in type I and type III collagen [13], increased expression of heat shock protein 70 (HSP70) [22]. More recent studies, particularly that of Cao *et al.* in 2011 [3], evaluated the effects of IPL on the biological and ultrastructural properties of fibroblasts in vitro after irradiation with increasing doses of IPL. These authors demonstrated an increase in cell viability and in the expression of type I and III procollagen mRNA and of transforming growth factor beta-1 (TGF-beta 1). A study on rats by Cho *et al.* [5] in 2012 showed an increase in collagen fibres and their diameter after 3 sessions of IPL with a 560 nm filter and a fluence of 30 J/cm^2. The increase in the diameter of the fibres did not depend on the number of applications of the handpiece but rather on the interval between the sessions (a longer interval of 3 weeks appears to be more favourable than a 1-week interval). Several clinical studies have confirmed these observations demonstrating an improvement in dermatoheliosis and skin texture. In 2002, Weiss *et al.* [23] assessed the long-term benefits of IPL treatment in 80 patients. After 4 years and an average of 3 treatments, improvements were noted in texture in 83% of patients, in telangiectasia in 82% of cases and in pigmentation in 79% of cases. In 2004, Sadick *et al.* [16] demonstrated improvement in wrinkles and solar elastosis in 93 patients with type I to III skin types 6 months after 5 treatment sessions spaced 4 weeks apart with an IPL Quantum (Lumenis) system. Bjerring *et al.* [2] assessed the use of 2 different wavelength bands (530-750 nm and 555-950 nm) in 20 patients and observed significant improvement in telangiectasia and pigmented lesions with the two types of filters (Ellipse DDD). More recently, biophysical measurements of human skin in an Asian study including 26 patients (chromametry for colour, cytometry for elasticity, visiometry for skin roughness, sebometry for seborrhea secretion and corneometry for hydration) seem to confirm the results of the other studies following 3 IPL sessions spaced 4 weeks apart: Shin *et al.* [17] demonstrated a more marked reduction in pigmentation after the first sessions for 84% of patients, improvements in elasticity and skin tone but a less significant reduction in wrinkles (although 58% of patients found their wrinkles to be improved). Sebum secretion and skin hydration remained unchanged. Other clinical studies report a reduction in pore size, improvement in skin texture and even a 2-year gain in age perception after each treatment session. As regards pigmentation lesions, the addition of a hydroquinone depigmenting agent increases the efficacy of IPL treatment [24], especially as hyperpigmentation may be observed after IPL treatment in cases of latent melasma, particularly in Asian patients [12].

Comparison between IPL and laser therapy

In 2006, Butler *et al.* [3] compared KTP laser therapy to IPL therapy in a split-face study in 17 patients with type I to IV skin types presenting pigmented and vascular lesions and/or discrete telangiectasia. The assessment at one month following one session showed improvement of the vascular and pigmented lesions with both techniques but patients reported more marked pain and oedema with KTP laser therapy. Treatment was nonetheless more rapid and more ergonomic with the laser. In 2008, Galeckas *et al.* [7] compared pulsed dye laser (PDL) with IPL in a split-face study of 10 patients. The results obtained after 3 treatment sessions spaced 3 to 4 weeks apart are shown in Tab. 2.

Table 2

Percentage of improvement	PDL	IPL
Dark lentigines	86.5%	82%
Light lentigines	65%	62.5%
Vessels < 0.6 mm	85%	78.5%
Vessels > 0.6 mm	38%	32.5%
Skin texture	40%	32%

For the patients, the improvement in vascular lesions was superior with PDL but treatment was also more painful. Tanghetti *et al.* [19] compared PDL with double band IPL therapy (500-670 and 870-1 200 nm) and reported similar efficacy and side effects after treating facial telangiectasia. Nymann *et al.* [14] compared the efficacy of a pulsed dye laser to that of an IPL device and demonstrated that both techniques were effective but the PDL was superior to IPL and caused less pain. Jorgensen *et al.* [8] assessed the efficacy and side effects of treatment with PDL and IPL after 6 months in a split-face study including 20 patients given 3 treatment sessions 3 weeks apart. They detected no significant differences in pigmentation or skin texture with the two methods, but found PDL to be more effective for telangiectasia. They found neither of the treatments effective for fine wrinkles but pain was more pronounced with IPL therapy. IPL alone does not seem to be very effective for the treatment of actinic keratosis and many authors try to optimize results by prior application of photosensitizing agents such as aminolevulinic acid (5-ALA) or *methyl aminolevulinate* (MAL).

Device settings

Filters filter out part of the rays given off by the lamp and define the medical indication. The spectral range is determined either by lower and higher wavelengths or by the colour of the filter filtering out the lower wavelengths (green, yellow, orange, red).

The adjusting of the pulse durations and the between-pulse periods varies depending on the devices and while experiences with various types of laser are more or less reproducible irrespective of the manufacturer, this is not so for IPL devices. Therefore, any publication providing information on IPL therapy should cite the brand and type of IPL device discussed in the article.

Nevertheless, general rules that may be adapted to any machine have been established for setting the devices depending on the target, see Tab. 3. In pigmented lesions, shorter wavelengths are absorbed more readily by melanin, which increases the risk of burns. For the treatment of patients with type I to III skin types, the usual wavelength settings (from 500 to 530 nm) can be used but exposure to the sun or UV light should be avoided. However, for the treatment of patients with type IV or higher skin types, the device should be more finely adjusted and fitted with stronger filters, fluence should be decreased and/or the time between the pulses and even between pulse repetitions should be increased. Pulse duration is short, between 2 and 10 ms (sometimes fractioned into 2 pulses). IPL does not lead to the fractioning of pigmented lesions unlike Q-switched lasers (closer to the thermal relaxation time of melanosomes which is between 50 and 280 ns). A fundamental study carried out in 2006 demonstrated the action of pulsed light on the basal layer melanosomes, which migrate towards the surface of the epidermis to be eliminated. The melanocytes of the lesions remain intact, their hyperactivity resumes after treatment. The authors concluded that pulsed light is effective for treating lesions with an increased number of melanosomes in the basal layer of the epidermis, but should be combined with a hydroquinone depigmenting agent or replaced by Q-switched laser irradiation in cases of melanocyte hyperactivity [26]. Higher wavelengths penetrate deeper into the skin and should be selected for the treatment of dermal pigmented lesions or deep-seated thick-walled vessels. Vascular lesions are treated by targeting haemoglobin, a chromophore contained in blood vessels whose 2 absorption peaks are 544 nm and 577 nm. It is easier to treat telangiectasia with IPL than diffuse erythrosis. Filters should be shorter for the treatment of fine vessels (500 nm) and slightly longer for the treatment of larger vessels (550 nm), which has the advantage of reducing absorption by the competitor chromophore, i.e. melanin. The finer the vessels, the shorter the pulse duration and the higher the fluence need to be. Higher filters are required for the treatment of thicker, blue vessels as well as pulse sequencing and longer periods between the pulses (longer treatment). Cooling systems protect the skin but reduce the efficacy of IPL if the vessels are fine.

Table 3

Colour of the filter	Green-yellow	Orange	Red-orange	Red
Wavelength	500/515	550	590	610
Depth	1 mm	2 mm	3 mm	4 mm
Vascular lesions	+++ Superficial fine vessels	+++ Deep vessels	+ Deep vessels	+/-
Pigmented lesions	+++ Risk of burns	++	+/-	+/-
Collagen remodelling	Superficial neocollagenesis	Neocollagenesis	Deep neocollagenesis	

Remodelling is achieved by stimulating fibroblast synthesis essentially via 2 routes: the vascular route with shorter wavelengths (release of vasoactive mediators by endothelial cells) and through a non-vascular heat effect with longer wavelengths (stimulation of heat shock proteins, of TGF-beta-1). This is translated by a tightening of the pores, enhanced tonus and improved elasticity, a more radiant complexion and an overall glow.

Treatment procedures

Several sessions are usually needed, typically around 2 to 6 depending on the degree of dermatoheliosis and the level of collagen stimulation required. They are spaced 4 to 6 weeks apart with annual or biannual maintenance sessions. The settings are selected based on which type of lesions is predominant (vascular or pigmented lesions) and the skin type of the patient. It is better to start with shorter wavelengths that are essentially absorbed by melanin and superficial vascular lesions and then once the skin has been lightened, the wavelengths and fluence may be increased to reach the deeper-lying lesions. Skin texture improvement is partially related to a heat effect, which is more marked during the first sessions when more chromophores are present, but the sessions may be repeated with a progressive increase of fluence to try to accentuate the improvements. A decrease in wrinkles and fine wrinkles should not be promised with IPL alone as stressed by several studies [6] because it is more the optical illusion of a radiant skin that gives the impression that the wrinkles are less deep according to the patients' self-assessments. Before each session, the skin must be perfectly cleansed and the eyes and cellular nevi protected. Coupling gel is applied in a thick layer over the whole of the area to be treated to enhance light transmission by decreasing the reflexion of light by the skin from 70 to 5%. No pressure should be exerted with the handpiece to avoid compressing the vessels. The spots, the average size of which is 5 cm^2 are made to overlap to avoid any irregularities. The pain is more intense with shorter wavelengths. With pigmented lesions, the clinical sign to look for is blackening, although this may not be very pronounced. Lesion blackening can take a few minutes. Little scabs generally form over 24 hours and disappear within about a week. Small-sized vessels generally disappear after treatment while medium-sized vessels become white or acquire a bluish tint before resuming their initial colour. They are eliminated after about a fortnight. The light needs to penetrate deeper for the treatment of larger vessels that are generally bluish or purplish. They become darker after treatment. Any erythema observed after the session disappears within a few hours. It is not unusual for oedemas that may be more pronounced under the eyes to be observed in the 2 to 3 days after the session if the skin is fine and dermatoheliosis is marked. The little scabs are more numerous with more pronounced pigmented lesions, giving the skin a "grimy" appearance for about 10 days Fig. 3, 4, but the application of an emollient cream and makeup is often sufficient to hide them. Makeup may be used immediately after the application of a moisturizing cream and patients may resume their activities without withdrawing from society. The use of topical depigmenting agents may be useful after the sessions.

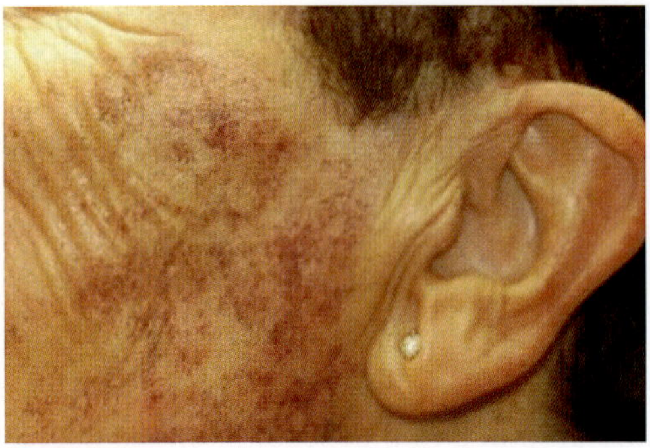

Figure 3 Scabby skin after a session
Spectral range: 530-750 nm
2 pulses of 2.5 ms separated by 10 ms – 8 joules

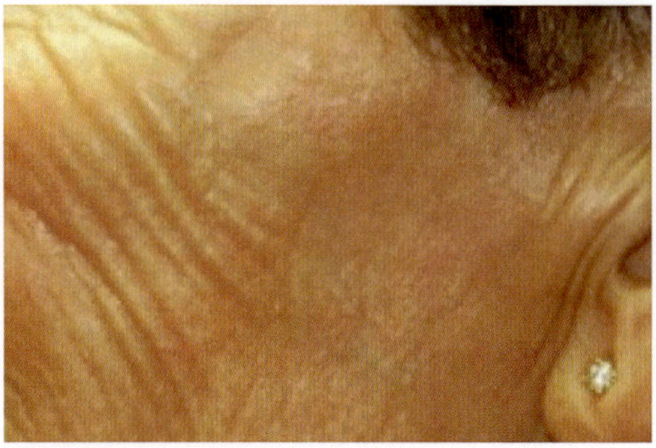

Figure 4 Results after a fortnight

Complications

Complications are often minimal and transient [15]. Erythema, which is common after a session, only lasts a few hours but may last longer if the skin is fine and reactive. Oedemas are also commonly observed in this type of skin and may persist for a few days. Treatment irregularities are easily corrected Fig. 5 with another session. Transient purpura may be observed with the shortest filters. Burns with blisters and scarring are observed only exceptionally when operators heed recommendations concerning skin type and pigmentation. They may give rise to hypo- or hyperpigmented scars, which generally grow fainter. Aggravation of vitiligo has also been described during treatment of areas other than the face [18]. Tattoos should not be treated and cellular nevi should be protected [21, 11]. Patients and operators are at a high risk of developing ocular lesions because the pigment of the iris absorbs light in the same wavelength range as that used with IPL [9].

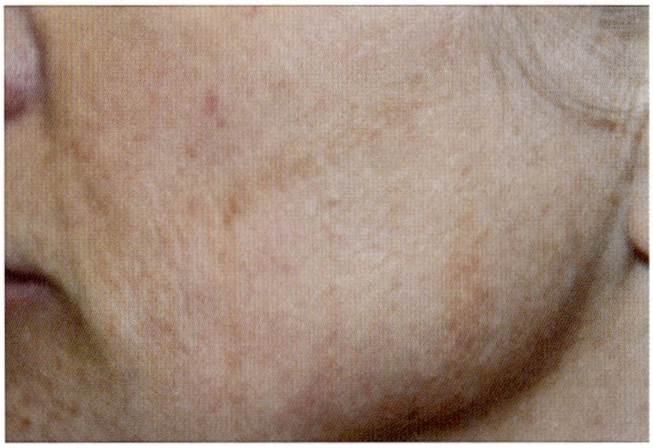

Figure 5 Treatment irregularities

IPL and photodynamic therapy

IPL may be used as a light source in photodynamic therapy (PDT). Either ALA or MAL at a concentration of 20% may be used as a photosensitizing agent and applied for period of 1 to 3 hours. Alternatively, a solution in the form of a spray [1] containing *liposome-encapsulated 0.5% 5-ALA to facilitate penetration may also be used. Published results report that efficacy is potentiated compared to use of light alone, especially for the treatment of pigmented lesions, fine wrinkles and actinic keratosis. However, the protocols are specific to each device because of differences in the spectral ranges used* [10]. The side effects are often comparable although the risk of post-inflammatory hyperpigmentation is higher [25].

CONCLUSION

Clinical results depend not only on the experience of the operator, but also largely on the quality of the IPL device which should be chosen with care since some devices are not sufficiently powerful or come with unsuitable filters that do not give appreciable results. However, recent technical improvements have allowed IPL therapy to gain a place in the therapeutic armamentarium against aging. Intense pulsed light is undeniably effective for the treatment of dermatoheliosis-related pigmented and vascular lesions and repeating the sessions improves skin texture and tone as well as illuminates the complexion. Repeating the sessions does not pose a problem given that patients may resume their normal activities immediately afterwards. Another non-negligible advantage of IPL therapy for freelance operators is that a single machine can be used for several purposes including hair removal, the treatment of inflammatory acne and scars or photodynamic therapy. Considering all the procedures available for the treatment of photoaging, it is logical that IPL should have a place among the first-line treatments.

The author would like to thank Mr D. Boutonnet for his help with the technical part of this chapter.

REFERENCES

[1] Bjerring P, Christiansen K, Troilius A, Bekhor P, de Leeuw J. Skin fluorescence controlled photodynamic photorejuvenation (wrinkle reduction). Laser Surg Med 2009; 41(5): 327-36.

[2] Bjerring P, Christiansen K, Troilius A, Diericks C. Facial photo rejuvenation using two different pulsed light wawelength bands. Lasers Surg Med 2004; 34: 120-6.

[3] Butler EG 2nd, McClellan SD, Ross EV. Split treatment of photodamaged skin with KTP 532 nm laser with 10 mm handpiece versus IPL: a cheek-to-cheek comparison. Lasers Surg Med 2006; 38(2): 124-8.

[4] Cao Y, Huo R, Feng Y, Li Q, Wang F. Effects of intense pulsed light on the biological properties and ultrastructure of skin dermal fibroblasts: potential roles in photoaging. Photomed Laser Surg 2011; 29(5): 327-32.

[5] Cho EB, Park H, Park EJ, Kwon IH, Kim SS, Kim KH, *et al.* Effect of intense pulsed light on rat skin. Dermatol Surg 2012; 38(3): 430-6.

[6] El-Domyati M, El-Ammawi TS, Moawad O, Medhat W, Mahoney MG, Uitto J. Intense pulsed light photorejuvenation: a histological and immunohistochemical evaluation. J Drugs Dermatol 2011; 10(11): 1246-52.

[7] Galeckas KJ, Collins M, Ross EV, Uebelhoer NS. Split-face treatment of facial dyschromia: pulsed dye laser with a compression handpiece versus intense pulsed light. Dermatol Surg 2008; 34(5): 672-80.
[8] Jørgensen GF, Hedelund L, Haedersdal M. Long-pulsed dye laser versus intense pulsed light for photodamaged skin: a randomized split-face trial with blinded response evaluation. Lasers Surg Med 2008; 40(5): 293-9.
[9] Lee WW, Murdock J, Albini TA, O'brien TP, Levine ML. Ocular damage secondary to intense pulse light therapy to the face. Ophthal Plast Reconstr Surg 2011; 27(4): 263-5.
[10] Maisch T, Moor AC, Regensburger J, Ortland C, Szeimies RM, Bäumler W. Intense pulse light and 5-ALA PDT: phototoxic effects in vitro depend on the spectral overlap with protoporphyrine IX but do not match cutoff filter notations. Lasers Surg Med 2011; 43(2): 176-82. doi: 10.1002/lsm.20970.
[11] Martín JM, Monteagudo C, Bella R, Reig I, Jordá E. Complete regression of a melanocytic nevus under intense pulsed light therapy for axillary hair removal in a cosmetic center. Dermatology 2012; 224(3): 193-7.
[12] Negishi K, Kushikata N, Takeuchi K, Tezuka Y, Wakamatsu S. Photorejuvenation by intense pulsed light with objective measurement of skin color in Japanese patients. Dermatol Surg 2006; 32(11): 1380-7.
[13] Negishi K, Wakamatsu S, Kushikata N, Tezuka Y, Kotani Y, Shiba K. Full-face photorejuvenation of photodamaged skin by intense pulsed light with integrated contact cooling: initial experiences in Asian patients. Lasers Surg Med 2002; 30(4): 298-305.
[14] TNymann P, Hedelund L, Haedersdal M. Long-pulsed dye laser vs. intense pulsed light for the treatment of facial telangiectasias: a randomized controlled trial. J Eur Acad Dermatol Venereol 2010; 24(2): 143-6.
[15] Radmanesh M, Azar-Beig M, Abtahian A, Naderi AH. Burning, paradoxical hypertrichosis, leukotrichia and folliculitis are four major complications of intense pulsed light hair removal therapy. J Dermatolog Treat 2008; 19(6): 360-3.
[16] Sadick NS, Weiss R, Kilmer S, Bitter P. Photorejuvenation with intense pulsed light: results of a multicenterstudy. J Drugs Dermatol 2004; 3(1): 41-9.
[17] Shin JW, Lee DH, Choi SY, Na JI, Park KC, Youn SW, *et al.* Objective and non-invasive evaluation of photorejuvenation effect with intense pulsed light treatment in Asian skin. J Eur Acad Dermatol Venereol 2011; 25(5): 516-22.
[18] Shin JU, Roh MR, Lee JH. Vitiligo following intense pulsed light treatment. J Dermatol 2010; 37(7):674-6.
[19] Tanghetti EA. Split-face randomized treatment of facial telangiectasia comparing pulsed dye laser and an intense pulsed light handpiece. Lasers Surg Med 2012; 44(2): 97-102.
[20] Trelles MA, Allones I, Velez M. Non-ablative facial skin photorejuvenation with an intense pulsed light system and adjunctive epidermal care. Lasers Med Sci 2003; 18(2):104-11.
22] Wang ML, Liu DL, Yuan Q. [Effect of intense pulsed light on heat shock protein 70 expression in skin]. Di Yi Jun Yi Da Xue Xue Bao. 2005; 25(1): 109-10.
[21] Weiss RA, Weiss MA, Beasley KL. Rejuvenation of photoaged skin: 5 years results with intense pulsed light of the face, neck, and chest. Dermatol Surg 2002; 28(12): 1115-9.
[22] Woodhall KE, Goldman MP, Gold MH, Biron J. Benefits of using a hydroquinone/tretinoin skin care system in patients undergoing intense pulsed light therapy for photorejuvenation: a placebo-controlled study. J Drugs Dermatol 2009; 8(9): 862-7.
[23] Xi Z, Shuxian Y, Zhong L, Hui Q, Yan W, Huilin D, Leihong X, Gold MH. Topical 5-aminolevulinic acid with intense pulsed light versus intense pulsed light for photodamage in Chinese patients. Dermatol Surg 2011; 37(1): 31-40.
[24] Yamashita T, Negishi K, *et al.* IPL therapy for superficial pigmented lesions evaluated by reflectance-mode confocal microscopy and optical coherence tomography. J Invest Dermatol 2006; 126: 2281-6.

CHAPTER 5

Skin resurfacing and conventional ablative lasers

Thierry Fusade

Photoablative laser resurfacing, also known as laser-abrasion, is a technique that is now quite old, since David made the first report of use of a pulsed CO_2 laser to resurface sun-damaged skin in 1989 [1]. Nonetheless, it remains the gold standard technique for many indications [2]. Though sometimes criticised for their downtime and risks of hypopigmentation, side effects are considerably reduced if patients are selected sensibly, a systematic technique is used, and post-operative follow-up is thorough.

PHYSICAL PRINCIPLES OF RESURFACING

The photoablative lasers used for resurfacing are CO_2 and Erbium:YAG lasers.

A 10,600 nm CO_2 laser is substantially absorbed by water, leading to a combination of vaporisation and diffusion of heat to the adjacent tissues. The 2,940 nm Erbium:YAG laser is the second type used in aesthetic resurfacing. It has a superior capacity for vaporisation due to its affinity for water, which is 10 to 20 times greater than that of the CO_2 laser. This difference means that at the wavelength usually used, Er:YAG has a greater ablative capacity and causes less heat diffusion. The photoablative mechanism is due to a very rapid energy transfer from the laser beam to the intra- or extra-cellular water, producing a sudden temperature increase to around 200-300° C. The sudden expansion caused by the vaporisation of this water is confined by the surrounding skin structures. Once the mechanical resistance capacity of the dermal collagen network is exceeded, the pressure generated induces the targeted tissue to explode and thus be eliminated.

The practice of resurfacing is based on an addition of several passes a photoablative laser causing the ablation of a specific cutaneous thickness in addition to the alteration of the tissue in contact with the ablation zone, due to the thermal effect. This means that with a CO_2 laser, given that the thermal relaxation time of the skin is 200-600 µs, a pulse duration of 1 ms limits thermal diffusion around the ablation zone to less than 100 μm. At that depth, the healing process cannot induce scars [3]. These values are different for the Erbium:YAG laser, which appears to have a much lower heat diffusion. It is for this reason that long-pulsed Erbium:YAG lasers have been developed. Producing pulse durations of around 10 ms, their effects can now rival those of the CO_2 laser [4].

CORRECTING DERMATOHELIOSIS THROUGH CUTANEOUS RESURFACING

The mechanisms involved in the process of dermatoheliosis correction are based on the combination of a number of phenomena.

– *The ablation* that the practitioner must restrict to the junction between the papillary dermis and the reticular dermis due to concerns for therapeutic safety.

– *The thermal effect* that induces denaturation of collagen bundles leading them to contract to as much as a quarter of their original length and to double in thickness.

– *The production of neocollagen* in the superficial and mid dermis as well as the reorganisation of the elastic fibre network.

When these events occur in association, this finally leads to smoothing out of wrinkles, homogenisation of the epidermis, renewed tightness, and dermal thickening as well as correction of elastosis [5]. The combination of these mechanisms is not the same for both the CO_2 laser and Erbium:YAG laser: at equivalent fluences, a greater number of passes is needed with the latter in order to achieve the same depth of ablation. Due to its more limited thermal effect, Er:YAG laser produces an inferior tightening effect, thus wrinkles are not corrected as well at the end of the post-operative remodelling phase. For this reason the short-pulsed Erbium:YAG laser appears to be more suitable for patients presenting only limited skin photodamage [6]. Currently, this laser proves to be a promising competitor for fractional ablative lasers when it is used in short-pulsed mode.

PATIENT SELECTION AND INFORMATION

Since the advent of both fractional ablative and non-ablative lasers, a rigorous process of patient selection, although already used, has become even more essential. Aesthetic resurfacing procedures must be restricted to patients with severe dermatoheliosis graded 3 or 4 on the Glogau scale.

Phototype

In principle, resurfacing can be performed on any skin type but the most severe cases of dermatoheliosis are seen in the lightest phototypes (phototype I-IV on the Fitzpatrick scale). In these circumstances, the vast majority of patients present a combination of dermal and epidermal lesions. Although resurfacing targets mainly lines and wrinkles, actinic keratosis and solar lentigines can also be reduced by abrasion of the epidermis. In parallel, vascular ectasia and dermal elastosis are also masked by the formation of neocollagen that is triggered.

Chosing the area to treat

In mild to moderate dermatoheliosis, it is entirely feasible to restrict treatment to one or two anatomical areas. However, for severe dermatoheliosis, the homogenisation of the skin complexion obtained by resurfacing makes it impossible to consider isolated treatment of a single area: the contrast between the treated and untreated areas would be even more visible on the untreated skin. This means that even if the patient's request concerns only one region (periorbital, perioral) it is sometimes difficult to avoid treating the whole face due to the extent of the photoinduced lesions, in order to favour an even result. In these cases, patients must be persuaded to reconsider their initial objectives and advised to undergo treatment of the whole face. Equally, any secondary hypopigmentation will be less obvious with full-face treatment [7]. Although it has been suggested, treatment of the neck and neckline should be avoided because of higher risk of scarring; the use of fractional lasers is preferred for these areas [8].

Identifying post-inflammatory hyperpigmentation risk

The patients that are at risk of developing post-inflammatory hyperpigmentation often have skin phototype III or higher, and they should also be identified during the initial consultation. In fact, patients have often already experienced this development after a prior inflammatory phenomenon. Predicting the occurrence of this hyperpigmentation means that the patient can be reassured about this benign and temporary side effect. In temperate regions resurfacing procedures should be avoided during the sunniest seasons or when there is less effective atmospheric filtration.

Medical contraindications

Some pre-existing medical conditions are a contraindication for aesthetic resurfacing. This is the case for a history of keloid or hypertrophic scarring, vitiligo, or psoriasis with the Koebner phenomenon [9]. Pathomimesis, problems with wound healing, and taking certain medications such as systemic corticosteroid therapy or isotretinoin in the six months prior to the intervention are also contraindications to this treatment.

Although not contraindications to the treatment, it is crucial to check for recurrent herpes infections, partially controlled diabetes, and any problems with haemostasis.

Identifying ectropion risk

If the lower eyelids are being treated, patients at risk of secondary ectropion are excluded. They can be identified based on two clinical features. A scleral show is mainly seen if there has been eyelid surgery prior to laser treatment. It can be assessed by asking the patient to open their mouth while looking upwards: if the lower eyelid detaches slightly from contact with the conjunctiva, this points to possible eyelid retraction after resurfacing. The same holds true for a positive snap-back test with the lower eyelid showing delayed return to contact with the eyeball when it is pinched between the fingers.

Patient information

Beyond clear instructions for patient selection, good compliance with the whole package of post-operative care entails providing the patient with detailed information about the chronology of the whole healing phase. It is important to explain to the patient that they will probably wish to exclude themselves socially for around two weeks, and subsequently women in particular will need to use make-up because of the residual erythema that will persist for between two and four months. Although the results can be spectacular, it needs to be emphasised that not all wrinkles will necessarily be completely removed, in order to avoid disappointment.

The patient should be told that, in contrast to misconstrued ideas, the moderate pain they experience will only occur while care is being carried out.

A quote and an informed consent form are given to the patient. These will be signed and returned at the second consultation when preoperative photographs will also be taken.

PERFORMING RESURFACING

Preventing herpes infection

Oral prevention of herpes infection (valaciclovir, famciclovir) is started at a preventive dose 24-48 hours before the intervention and will be continued throughout the re-epithelialisation phase. While some practitioners recommend routine anti-viral treatment, others restrict this to patients with a history of recurrent herpes infection. There is a lack of consensus over the duration of anti-herpes cover: recommendations vary from the first five days post-operatively to the whole of the healing phase [10, 11].

Facial resurfacing

Full-face resurfacing is carried out under general anaesthesia: it is almost impossible to achieve full and comfortable desensitisation of the face through a combination of nerve blocks and anaesthetic creams. Pre-operatively the patient will have been shampooed using a foaming antiseptic solution and undergone total disinfection of the face. Landmarks will be made with a dermographic pen while the patient is standing in order to determine the position of the mandibular border as well as the border between the orbital regions and adjacent jugular-temporal regions.

The treatment is then carried out by working on each anatomic unit one after the other. To treat a wrinkle, the cutaneous part adjacent to the furrow must be smoothed: it is by blending these two edges that a satisfactory result can be obtained. There are two possible ways to proceed with resurfacing. Either the first step is a pass over the edges of the most significant wrinkles before a second overall pass is made, or the approach is the reverse with an initial full pass being carried out before the second pass is performed over the wrinkles that are still visible. Depending on the locations, a third pass may be performed, especially on the anterior part of the cheeks or the glabella. In terms of clinical features, each consecutive pass performed during resurfacing will target the epidermis successively, which will whiten and separate with a crinkled appearance under the thermal effect of the CO_2 laser, or will be broken down into fine debris with the Erbium:YAG laser. The treated surface is cleaned immediately using a gauze or cotton bud soaked with sterile saline solution. This step has proven to be crucial in order to avoid the debris that remains in place absorbing the laser beam, which could create focused points of heat or generate a masking effect making the second pass uneven. Once cleaned, the superficial dermis is exposed and is an even pinkish colour. During the second pass, the skin takes on a whitish colour and it contracts if treated by CO_2 laser. Short-pulsed Erbium:YAG laser, by contrast, induces mild suffusion haemorrhage. The use of a "long" Erbium:YAG laser produces an appearance similar to that obtained with CO_2 laser. With both of these laser treatments, a third pass over some areas is possible, such as the midline of the forehead or anterior cheek as this will optimise the tightening effect Fig. 1.

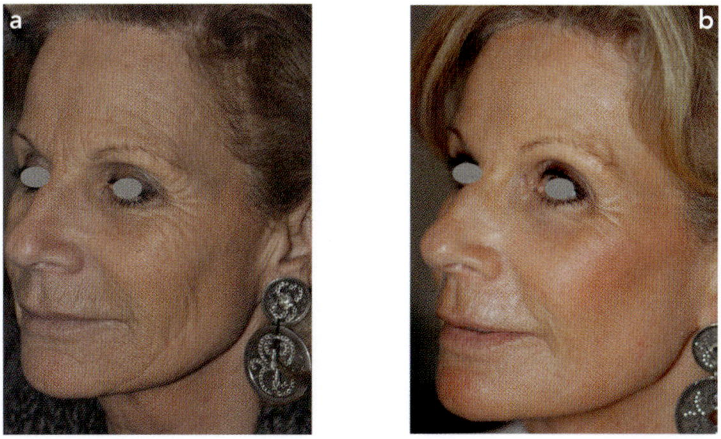

Figure 1 Full-face resurfacing with pulsed CO_2 laser
Before treatment (a), result at 6 months (b)

Resurfacing an anatomic unit

Regional aesthetic resurfacing can essentially be practised on three anatomic units Fig. 2-4: the upper lip, the lower lip and chin, and the periorbital region. For these treatments local anaesthetic can be offered. In order to avoid a marked contrast with

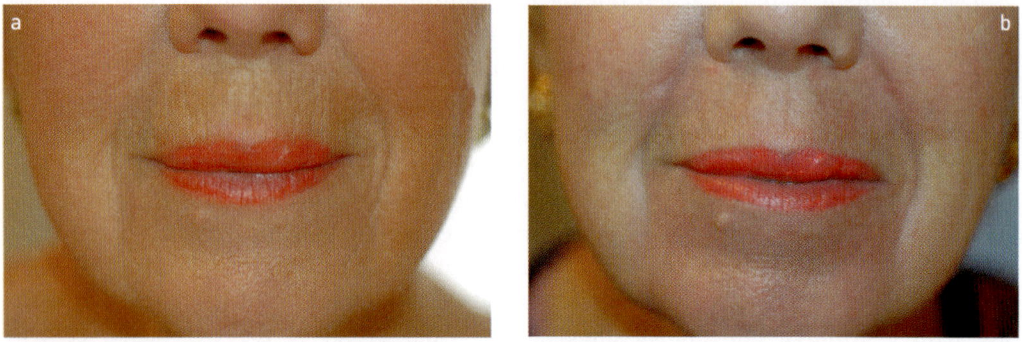

Figure 2 **Upper lip resurfacing with pulsed CO_2 laser**
Before treatment (a), result at 6 months (b)

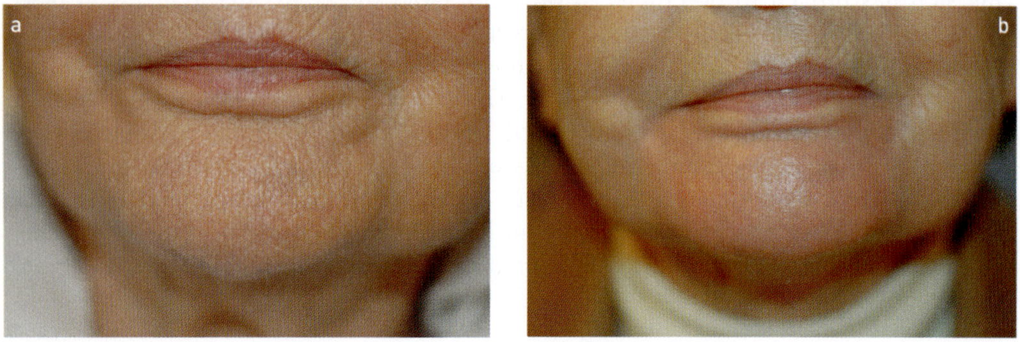

Figure 3 **Correction of elastosis of the chin by CO_2 laser resurfacing**
Before treatment (a), result at 3 months (b)

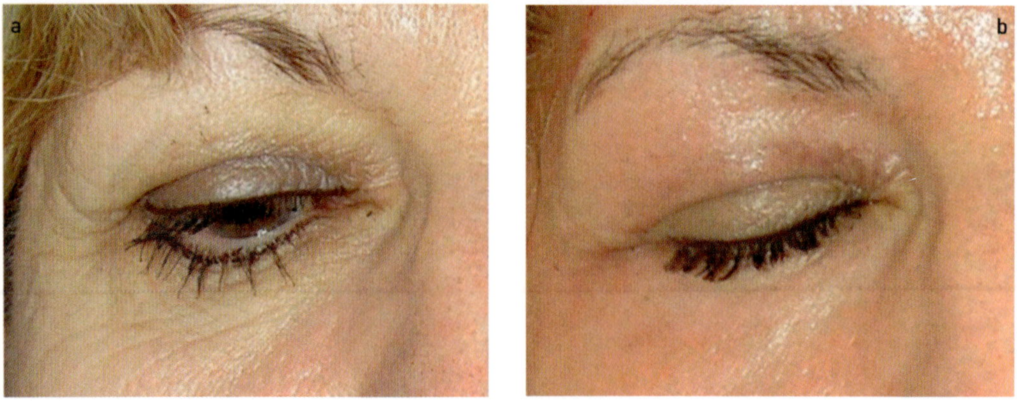

Figure 4 **Periorbital resurfacing**
Before treatment (a), result at 3 months (b)

untreated adjacent regions, candidates must present only moderate actinic epidermal lesions. If not, the procedure could be completed by a TCA skin peel on the areas left untreated by laser [2].

When treating these areas, it is more straightforward to perform the initial pass over the shoulders of the wrinkles and then a second overall pass. No more than two passes may be carried out over the lower eyelid, but a third pass may be performed on the perioral unit targeting the vermilion border.

POST-OPERATIVE FOLLOW-UP

Post-operative care

There are two opposing techniques used: an "open" or "closed" wound care system. The terms open and closed describe whether the dermal abrasions are covered with occlusive dressings or not. The need to use lipid phase occlusive topical treatments in order to maintain a hydrophobic film that forms a substitute protective barrier is still recognised: pure white petrolatum, ointments consisting of a mix of petrolatum and lanolin alcohol, or silicone-based topical treatments. The predominantly aqueous phase of creams does not seem to ensure prolonged occlusion; they must therefore be avoided in our opinion. It is possible to use an antibiotic ointment for prophylaxis on the zones that have undergone abrasion but this can be poorly tolerated and it is not essential if the dressings are applied with a rigorous approach to antisepsis. These ointments remain useful for the orifices close to the treated area: nostrils, external auditory canals.

In practice, closed wound care must be carried out twice daily during the phase when residual debris and wound exudates are being eliminated. It is then a daily process until re-epithelialisation is complete. The dressings are changed after having been moistened with sterile isotonic saline solution. The skin that has undergone abrasion is cleaned using sterile saline or antiseptic solution, and then the petrolatum-based emollient is applied in a thick layer in order to avoid the dressings subsequently adhering to the area. At the same time, a local antibiotic is applied to the nearby orifices. The dressing is then closed using non-woven gauzes held in place by medical tape or surgical mesh. For an open wound care system, full cleansing is carried out in the morning and evening; in the interval, a petrolatum-based emollient is applied every two to three hours [12]. It does nonetheless seem to be difficult to continue this care without using gauzes as protection during the night given the discomfort that wounds can cause during sleep. In all cases, care must be continued until re-epithelialisation is complete. The adhesive semi-permeable membrane dressings that were in the past much more commonly used have been progressively abandoned due to the risk of secondary infection [13].

Functional signs

In the days following the treatment, pain is reduced by the occlusive care. It is a similar sensation to sunburn for the first two or three days, which then changes to pruritus and a pulling sensation that continues for several weeks. There may be oedema to the eyelid that can sometimes be significant, meaning that it is unable to open, especially after CO_2 laser.

Post-operative outcome

Re-epithelialisation of the areas treated with abrasion varies depending on the type of laser used, the depth of the abrasion, and the area treated. The process lasts between ten and twelve days when the treatment has been carried out using an Erbium:YAG laser, and it can be as long as around two weeks with a pulsed CO_2 laser. If wound healing in aesthetic resurfacing exceeds around two weeks, this must alert the practitioner to the possibility of abnormal scarring (see below). When the cutaneous barrier is re-established, the skin remains erythematous, as epidermal maturation is still modest. For a period of several weeks, linear purpuric striae may develop at the slightest rubbing. In practical terms, it is essential to also advise the patient to avoid wearing rings and bracelets as they can cause microtraumas by rubbing during sleep. Milia can appear during epithelialisation. They regress spontaneously in a few weeks [9]. Persistent erythema fades away over a period of 2-4 months with the Erbium:YAG laser and 4-6 months with the CO_2 laser Fig. 5 and 6. During this time, it is crucial to wear sunscreen in order to prevent post-inflammatory hyperpigmentation [14]. The periorbital region is protected by wearing sunglasses with a wide frame and lenses with a high filtration capacity.

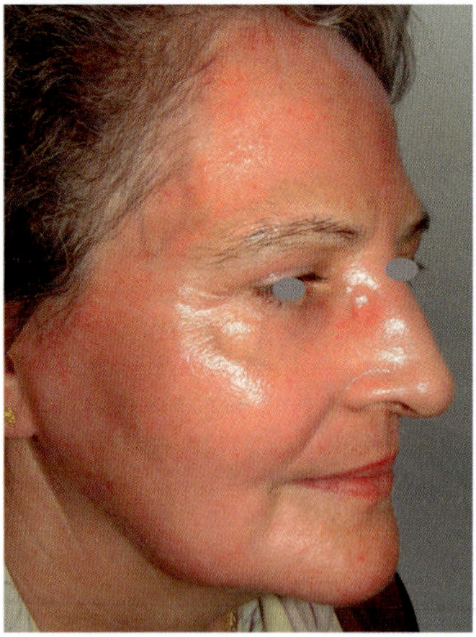

Figure 5 Facial resurfacing, result at 21 days

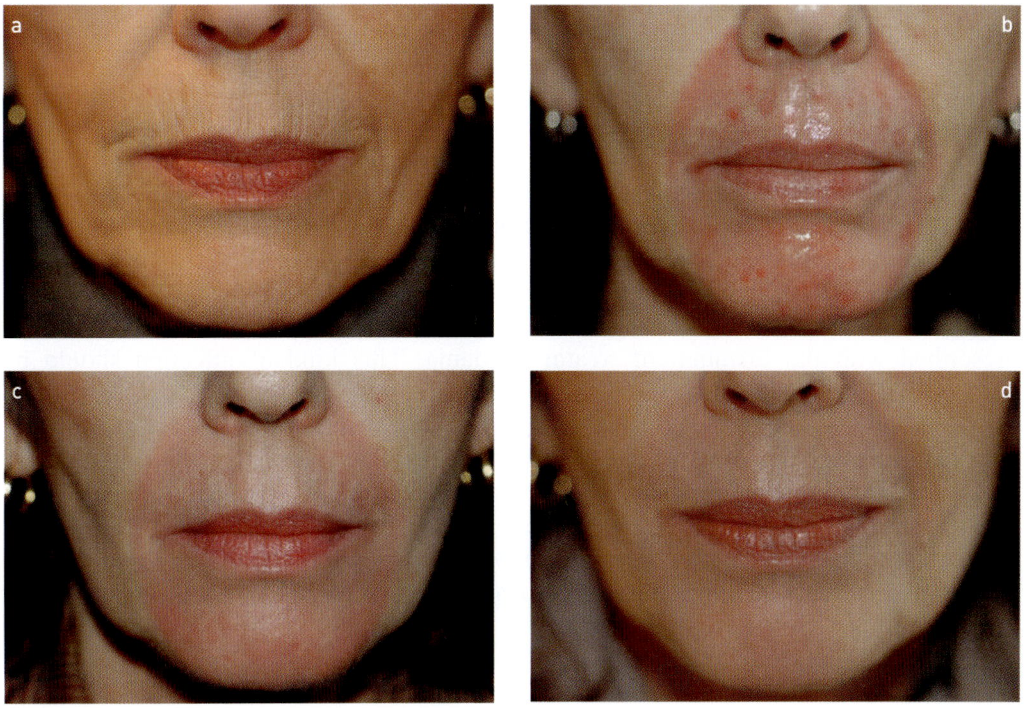

Figure 6 Chronology of healing
A D0 (a), at D12 (b), at D21 (c) and at D60 (d)

RESULTS

While a very clear improvement in dermatoheliosis is obtained after resurfacing in all patients, the extent of this improvement varies between cases and by region treated. The benefit that can be expected on photoinduced fine lines has proven excellent, but dynamic wrinkles that are triggered by facial muscle contraction tend to gradually reappear as the years go by. A retrospective study has demonstrated in this respect that improved skin texture is maintained in 32% and 20% of patients at 5 and 10 years after CO_2 laser resurfacing but that wrinkles reappear in 88% and 98% of patients respectively in the same timeframes [7]. A protocol that also uses adjuvant treatments a few months after resurfacing leads to longer-lasting results. With this in mind, other treatments to offer could be botulinum toxin treatment to the forehead, crows' feet, or lower eyelids, or perhaps redefining the lip outline with hyaluronic acid, an excellent supporting procedure that limits the reappearance of radial wrinkles.

SIDE EFFECTS

Infectious complications

During the healing phase, extensive herpes in the areas treated with abrasion is a worrying complication as it can lead to scars [9]. It is treated with an anti-herpes virus agent at a curative dose taken orally or even via the parenteral route. A secondary bacterial or yeast infection can also occur. The risk of this may have been increased in the past due to usage of systemic corticosteroids that were sometimes prescribed with the intention of treating oedema. This kind of infection should be suspected if the patient presents persistent pain, burning or fever, or purulent deposits or pustules at the peripheries of the areas treated with abrasion. A bacterial infection requires oral treatment with an antibiotic effective on staphylococcus and will then be adjusted depending on the results from bacteriology specimens. A secondary infection with candidiasis needs to be treated with fluconazole. Routine use of antiseptics during wound care in combination with careful hand washing followed by the use of hydro-alcoholic antiseptic gels considerably limits these kinds of secondary infections.

Persistent erythema and hypopigmentation

While post-healing erythema is normal and must be explained clearly to the patient, it often indicates that the abrasion was too deep if it persists after six months: it is then common that it gives way to hypopigmented skin. This hypopigmentation corresponds to the destruction of melanocytes at the dermo-epidermal junction and also in follicle reservoirs. Use of an excimer laser can sometimes produce secondary repigmentation of hypopigmented areas by mobilising melanocytes from extra-follicular reservoirs Fig. 7. A retrospective study with a 10-year follow-up of patients who had undergone CO_2 laser resurfacing found hypopigmentation in 8.7% of patients at the end of this period [7].

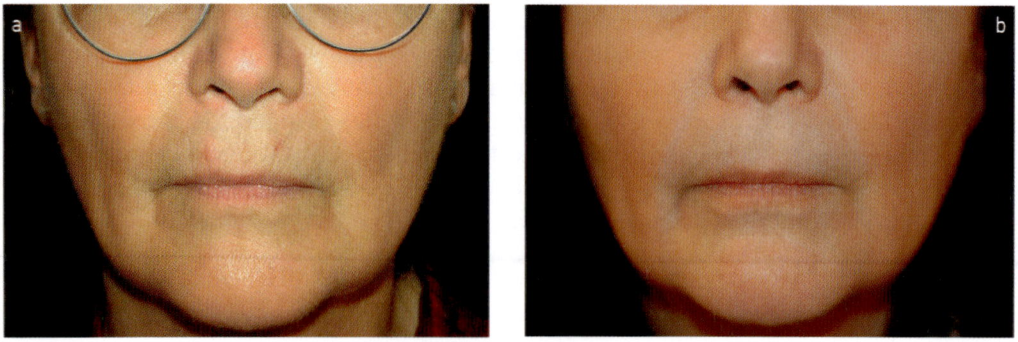

Figure 7 Side effect, persistent hypopigmentation
Before treatment (a), persistent hypopigmentation 4 years after perioral CO_2 laser resurfacing (b)

Post-inflammatory hyperpigmentation

This is more common in subjects with higher phototypes but it does sometimes occur in lighter phototypes. Although favoured by UV rays, even daylight without sun exposure can be enough to trigger it. In all cases, it is treated with a combination of sunscreen to avoid aggravation and daily gentle topical skin lightening treatments from the end of the first month after the intervention. If symptoms persist, Kligman's trio can be offered with caution from the third month.

Abnormal scarring

True hypertrophic scars indicate that the abrasion procedure was poorly controlled or too deep [9] Fig. 8. They mainly arise on areas of high mobility such as the perioral region or the corners of the jaw. Compression treatment using suitable dressings possibly later combined with pulsed dye laser treatment or corticosteroid injections will bring them to an end but not without sequelae of further scars.

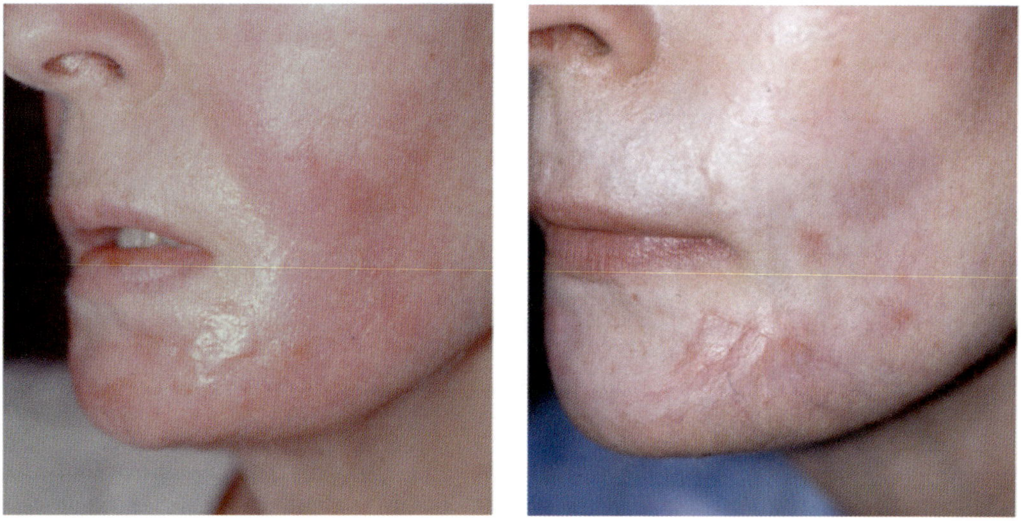

Figure 8 Side effect, hypertrophic scars induced by CO_2 laser resurfacing that was too deep

Ectropion

Ectropion is a complication that may appear after lower eyelid resurfacing. Once again, it is caused by an abrasion that was too aggressive or carried out on an already-tightened lower eyelid. If it was not possible to identify the risk when the patient was selected, it is necessary to suggest regular massage of the eyelid once healing has been achieved. The retraction, in a similar way to hypertrophic scarring, often regresses in a few weeks. If it does persist, only a later surgical intervention is able to correct it.

CONCLUSION

Resurfacing using conventional photoablative lasers is still the treatment of choice to offer to patients for severe dermatoheliosis. Only a rigorous patient selection process, full and clear explanation of the aftermath, and attentive practice of the post-resurfacing care and treatment (not neglecting the crucial post-operative support), can guarantee that the treatment is accepted without any adverse memories for the candidate.

REFERENCES

[1] David LM, Lask GP, Glassberg E, Jacoby R, Abergel RP. Laser abrasion for cosmetic and medical treatment of facial actinic damage. Cutis 1989; 43(6): 583-587.

[2] Sandel HD 4th, Perkins SW. CO_2 laser resurfacing: still a good treatment. Aesthet Surg J 2008; 28 (4): 456-462.

[3] Ross EV, Domankevitz Y, Skrobal M, Anderson RR. Effects of CO_2 laser pulse duration in ablation and residual thermal damage: implications for skin resurfacing. Lasers Surg Med 1996; 19(2): 123-129.

[4] Trelles MA, Mordon S, Benítez V, Levy JL. Er:YAG laser resurfacing using combined ablation and coagulation modes. Dermatol Surg 2001; 27(8): 727-734.

[5] Lessa S, Nanci M, Flores E. Histologic study of the structural changes in fine palpebral skin following selective photothermolysis with CO_2 laser. Aesthetic Plast Surg 2009; 33(1): 66-71.

[6] Alster TS, Lupton JR. Erbium:YAG cutaneous laser resurfacing. Dermatol Clin 2001; 19(3): 453-466.

[7] Prado A, Andrades P, Danilla S, Benitez S, Reyes S, Valenzuela G, Guridi R, Fuentes P. Full-face carbon dioxide laser resurfacing: a 10-year follow-up descriptive study. Plast Reconstr Surg 2008; 121(3): 983-993.

[8] Kilmer SL, Chotzen VA, Silva SK, McClaren ML. Safe and effective carbon dioxide laser skin resurfacing of the neck. Lasers Surg Med 2006; 38(7): 653-657.

[9] Nanni CA, Alster TS. Complications of carbon dioxide laser resurfacing. An evaluation of 500 patients. Dermatol Surg 1998; 24(3): 315-320.

[10] Bisaccia E, Scarborough D. Herpes simplex virus prophylaxis with famciclovir in patients undergoing aesthetic facial CO_2 laser resurfacing. Cutis 2003; 72(4): 327-328.

[11] Beeson WH, Rachel JD. Valacyclovir prophylaxis for herpes simplex virus infection or infection recurrence following laser skin resurfacing. Dermatol Surg 2002; 28(4): 331-336.

[12] Atiyeh BS, Dham R, Costagliola M, Al-Amm CA, Belhaouari L. Moist exposed therapy: an effective and valid alternative to occlusive dressings for post laser resurfacing wound care. Dermatol Surg 2004; 30(1): 18-25.

[13] Christian MM, Behroozan DS, Moy RL. Delayed infections following full-face CO_2 laser resurfacing and occlusive dressing use. Dermatol Surg 2000; 26(1): 32-36.

[14] Hedelund L, Haedersdal M, Egekvist H, Heidenheim M, Hans CW, Poulsen T. CO_2 laser-resurfacing: increased risk of side effects after uv-exposure: an experimental animal study. Lasers Surg Med 2005; 36(2): 79-84.

CHAPTER 6

Facial aging and non-ablative fractional photothermolysis

Hans Laubach, Bertrand Pusel

INTRODUCTION

It is well established that traditional skin resurfacing techniques using ablative and non-ablative lasers can improve the appearance of the aging skin [1, 2]. However, patients are more and more reticent about accepting the side effects and risks associated with traditional ablative resurfacing techniques [3]. In addition, the results obtained with traditional non-ablative laser techniques (1,320 nm Nd:YAG lasers, pulsed dye lasers as well as 1,450 and 1,540 nm laser resurfacing) are inconsistent and hence often unpredictable [4, 5].

To overcome the drawbacks related to these techniques, Manstein *et al.* [6] developed the concept of fractional photothermolysis (FP) in 2004. Fractional photothermolysis creates arrays of microscopic thermal injuries called Microscopic Treatment Zones (MTZs) measuring less than 200 micrometer in diameter. Since the surrounding skin remains unharmed the intact epidermal cells can be recruited for a rapid healing of the MTZs in less than 24 hours [7]. The term “fractional photothermolysis” has been coined to indicate that only a small fraction and not the entire surface area is directly exposed to the laser.

Non-ablative fractional photothermolysis (nFP) is an effective method for treating a number of clinical signs of facial aging. It has an effect not only on fine wrinkles and skin texture but also on dyspigmentation and telangiectasia.

TECHNICAL ASPECTS

Near infrared laser wavelengths can be used for nFP since their chromophore is mostly water and hence the penetration is independent of other chromophores like melanin and hemoglobine. The specificity of the FP concept is that the MTZs are small enough (in general less than 200 micrometer in diameter) that the damaged or destroyed epidermis may be repaired within one or two days and at the same time not causing permanent dermal fibrosis.

MTZs within the skin generated by the FP treatment can also be seen as the first way of a three dimensional treatment approach of the skin. MTZs are shaped either like inverted cones or tapered columns and they can extend more or less deeply into the dermis. The degree of thermal damage within an MTZ is generally sufficient in the case of non-ablative FP to cause cell necrosis and collagen coagulation and in the case of ablative FP additional thermal tissue ablation. Because of the proximity of keratinocytes in the non-treated area, the epidermis can be restored a few hours after the treatment. In the case of nFP even the skin barrier function is preserved at all times since the *stratum corneum* does not contain sufficient water to be thermally destroyed and hence remains intact (this is not the case for the more invasive form of ablative FP). This was demonstrated by Manstein et al. who showed no significant changes in trans-epidermal water loss after nFP [6]. Histological observation during the days following a FP procedure showed, that small epidermal particles called Microscopic Epidermal Necrotic Debris (MENDs) migrate towards the surface of the epidermis. Their subsequent upward migration and shedding is due to the migration of unharmed keratinocytes from the surrounding area into the epidermal MTZ. Clinically this can be seen as slight brown desquamation Fig. 1. It takes one week for all the MENDs to be released and the epidermis to appear normal again on histopathological examination [7]. Histochemical studies with specific staining have shown that MENDs are composed of epidermal debris

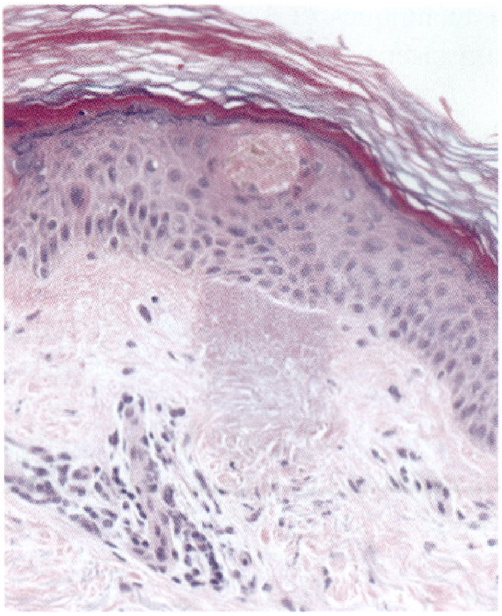

Figure 1 Histology one day after treatment

but may also, surprisingly, include portions of dermal tissue. The process of release of dermal and epidermal debris by nFP is generally referred to as the MEND-shuttle [8].

While epidermal damage heals rapidly, the dermal portions of MTZs are still present weeks and months after the procedure. These dermal MTZs are visible as columns of collagen coagulation surrounded by various amounts of inflammatory infiltrates. It takes three months for the dermal portions of the MTZs to no longer be evidenced by routine histological examinations [9]. In summary nFP produces microscopically small areas (MTZs) of thermally necrotized tissue epidermal and dermal tissue in the shape of inverted cones while preserving the *stratum corneum*.

CHOICE OF TREATMENT PARAMETERS

Certain basic treatment rules should be taken into account when selecting the nFP parameters.

First, laser focusing and fluence should be selected to keep the diameter of the MTZs in the sub-millimeter range ultimately enabling epidermal regeneration within a few hours Fig. 2. Another advantage associated with this microscopic diameter of each MTZ is that the lesions are so small that they cannot be seen with the naked eye, guaranteeing a homogeneous appearance of the treatment area at all the times after the treatment. The depth of the MTZs, however, may extend even several millimetres down into the deep dermis without precluding rapid and scar-free healing of the treated area as long as the diameter stays in the sub-millimeter range.

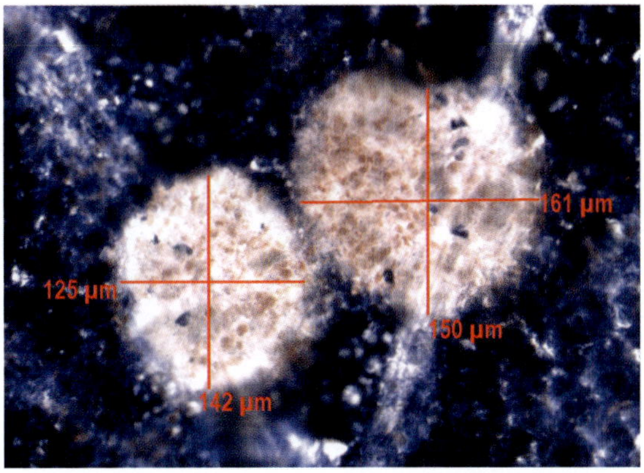

Figure 2 Diameter of the MTZs

Secondly, sufficient healthy skin must be left between the MTZs to allow for sufficient tissue repair capability and epidermal adherence. In non-ablative fractional photothermolysis, all the energy delivered to the tissues is transformed into heat. Therefore unheated skin areas in between the MTZs are necessary to avoid the loss of thermal confinement of the heat injury resulting in bulk heating of the entire dermis. It is due to the significant depth of the MTZs possibly reaching the deeper dermis that this type of excessive tissue heating may ultimately result in thermal damage similar to that observed in third-degree burns. Another mechanism to avoid bulk-heating is to allow for sufficiently long time intervals in between consecutive treatment passes to allow tissue cooling before a subsequent pass. Additionally, external skin cooling does help to reduce the accumulation of heat in the treated area and is at the same time useful to reduce treatment associated pain.

To chose the desired amount of skin surface treated, two separate techniques are used to generate the necessary density of MTZs (number of MTZs per unit of area), i.e. the "stamping" and the "rolling" technique. It seems that neither technique is ideal. It is the authors experience that the "rolling" technique enables the quicker and more homogenous treatment of larger surfaces areas whereas the "stamping" technique is more suitable for the treatment of areas with an irregular surface profile. With both techniques, the final total density of MTZs and with this the treated surface area may be easily adjusted by changing the number of treatment passes. Ideally the MTZ density should be decreased on the margins of a treated area to avoid demarcation lines between treated and untreated areas, another feature unique to the concept of FP.

All in all, it is best to choose the treatment parameters (particularly fluence/MTZ and MTZ-density) as a function of the particular treatment indication and each patient's desire to assure that the results and postoperative care are conform to both the practitioner's and patient's expectations.

INDICATIONS

Non-ablative fractional lasers have been shown to be effective for the management of various conditions including aging of facial and other areas of the skin, as well as for the treatment of acne scars, all types of atrophic scars, actinic keratosis and certain pigment disorders. There have also been anecdotal reports of them being useful for the treatment of involutive hemangiomas, granuloma annulare, minocycline-induced pigmentation and other types of skin diseases [1, 3, 10].

PATIENT SELECTION

A preoperative visit is similar to most procedures mandatory and the patient's informed consent has to be obtained before the treatment. During this first visit, the entire medical history, especially prior plastic surgery interventions, should be assessed and a thorough medical examination should be performed. Especially the treatment area requires meticulous clinical examination to check for any concurrent suspect lesion that may need to be biopsied before the procedure.

Similarly, the patient's skin type should be recorded in the medical record as patients with darker skin types are at higher risk of postoperative hyperpigmentation. Any contraindications to treatment with nFP should also be excluded during the visit. Contraindications essentially include treatment with isotretinoin or isotretinoin treatment discontinued less than 6 months ago, progressive dermatitis in the treatment area and, to a lesser extent, a history of keloid scars and, as a precaution, pregnancy. The purpose of the visit is furthermore to ensure that the patient's expectations can be met by the nFP technique, particularly as the results are generally only visible at a later stage, at least 3 to 6 months after the treatment.

Treatment modalities vary from one device to another but it is generally agreed upon that satisfactory results can be obtained with 3 to 5 sessions spaced at least 15 days apart. Although patient satisfaction appears to be correlated with the number of sessions, the additional benefit in between the third and subsequent sessions seems to be marginal [11]. Standardized photography should be performed for all patients before and after the treatment. Furtermore, in our practice, all patients systematically receive prophylactic antiviral medication for herpes simplex infection 2 days before laser treatment. In addition all patients should be made aware of the importance of strict sun protection for several months depending on the degree of the induced skin inflammation. Finally, patients should also already receive a prescription with detailed instructions for all products required during the postoperative period.

WHAT OCCURS DURING A SESSION?

At first all makeup should be removed and the skin should be cleansed and wiped with a 70% isopropyl alcohol solution. If required, the treatment area can be anesthetised by different anaesthetic creams (incubation time in general > 1 hour). For this purpose different products containing lidocaine and prilocaine are available but for all of these products the recommended precautions must be kept in mind to avoid any local side effects, especially corneal erosions by accidental contact with the eye, and also potential systemic toxicity. For this reason the area to be treated should not exceed 300 to 400 cm^2. After the incubation period of the topical anaesthetic cream it should be removed entirely. The patients eyes should then be protected with appropriate eye protection for the laser treatment and laser safety googles should be handed to all the other people in the treatment room.

The laser session includes a variable number of passes over the treatment area based on the desired final density (MTZ/cm^2) as described previously. During the treatment patients typically report stinging combined with a more or less acute sensation of heat. Therefore, depending on the device, adjunctive analgesia using forced air cooling may be useful to improve patient comfort. Post treatment effects include transient moderate erythema (100% of patients) and very frequent oedema (particularly in zones with reduced dermal thickness like the periorbital area), prolonged by a "sunburn" effect and mild desquamation lasting 3 to 5 days on average. Most patients also complain about dry skin and varying degrees of skin sensitivity [12]. To reduce the severity of these side effects postoperative care including the use of vaporized spring water and the application of soothing moisturizing creams can be started immediately after the treatment session. Patients should continue to use a mosturizing cream ideally in combination with gentle skin cleansing and the frequent application of high SPF 50 sunscreen several days after the treatment. In addition patients should be warned to avoid any rubbing of the treated area because of the increased fragility of the epidermal-dermal attachement and the increased risk of epidermlysis following nFP treatment. Patients presenting with a particular risk of post-inflammatory hyperpigmentation (PIH) may be prescribed topical dermocorticosteroids. Since the best treatment for any medical disease or side effect remains its prevention treatment parameters, especially energy/MTZ and density, should be chosen and adjusted prudently and with great care.

CLINICAL RESULTS

Non-ablative fractional photothermolysis has been demonstrated to be effective for a wide variety of conditions where collagen remodelling is required for example for the treatment of fine to moderate wrinkles. Treatment of wrinkles and crow's feet was also the first indication recognized for nFP by the FDA in the United States. Manstein's first publication in 2004 [6] was rapidly confirmed by other authors [13, 14]. Contrary to the results obtained with botulinum toxin or dermal filler products, the results obtained with nFP are based on neocollagenesis and therefore persist over time. Additionally, the technique is not associated with the risk of overcorrection as it is based on a natural process. NFP however shows only very limited efficacy in the treatment of deep facial wrinkles such as the vertical wrinkles above the upper lip. Nevertheless nFP has an important place in the overall management of mild to moderate changes of the aging skin Fig. 3 and Fig. 4.

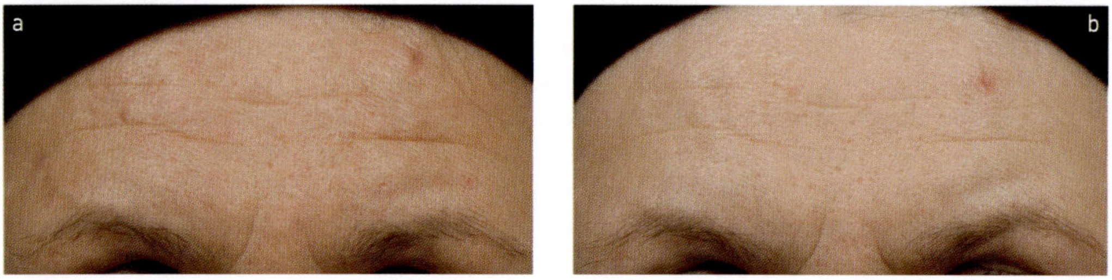

Figure 3 Treatment of forehead wrinkles at D0 (a) and at 6 months (b)

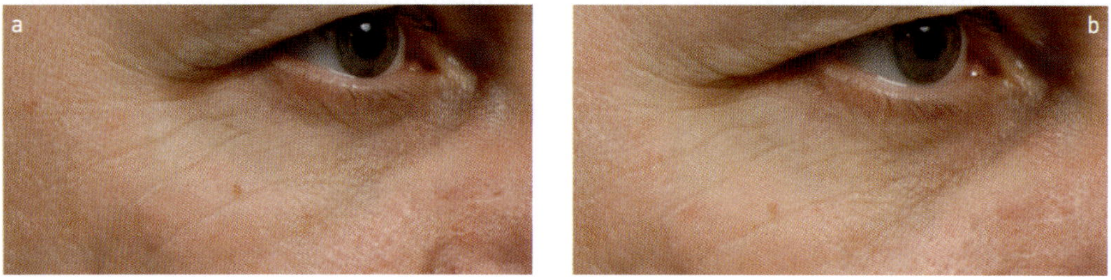

Figure 4 Treatment of periorbital wrinkles at D0 (a) and at 6 months (b)

Concerning the optimal number of treatment sessions 3 to 5 sessions with nFP are required to guarantee acceptable clinical improvement but the optimal number of treatment session is disputed and remains controversial. Although it is consistently agreed that several treatment sessions improve results, it is not known exactly how the number of treatment sessions is related to overall improvement in specific indications. The complexity of nFP and the numerous choices that need to be made by the operator partially explain the lack of clinical studies comparing the various FP-specific parameters on the final results.

With the aim of optimizing treatment parameters, Peukert [15] investigated treatment efficacy in a study with a splitface design. One side of the patients' faces was treated with high density and low energy/MTZs and the other side of their faces were treated with low density and high energy/MTZs. However the total energy used for each facial side was equal for both sides of the face just differently distributed. Significant improvement was obtained on both sides. Clinical results were slightly better with the use of higher energy/MTZ settings, but these settings were correlated with intense erythema and oedema, sometimes lasting more than a week resulting in important social down-time for the patient. The use of low energy/MTZ settings only gave rise to an erythema for 2 to 3 days combined with the near absence of oedeme Fig. 5.

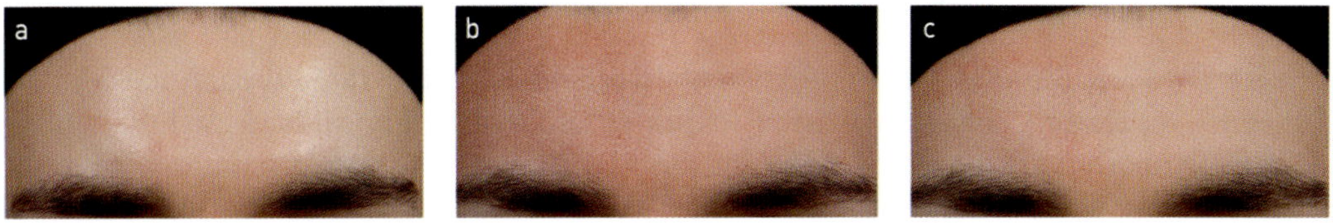

Figure 5 Side effects on D0 (a), D2 (b) and D5 (c)
Splitface treatment with the right side treated with high density/low energy/MTZs and the left side treated with low density/high energy/MTZs, keeping total energy input for each facial side constant

It should be mentioned once more that one of the physician's obligations is the patient's education in order to assure that their expectations regarding efficacy and side effects are realistic and reasonable.

The 1,550 nm fiber laser developed in 2006 is the device that has been by far studied the most. It can deliver energies/MTZ in between 4 and 70 mJ and reaches a maximum MTZ depth with the 70 mJ setting of about 1,400 µm with either a 5 mm or 15 mm handpiece. The total skin area covered by MTZs in relation to the remaining healthy skin (fill factor) is chosen typically in between 4 and 48% and determined by the number of passes and the diameter of each MTZ. All these parameters can and should be adjusted by the operator as a function of the selected indication and the skin type of the patient.

Aditionally, the nFP 1,550 nm laser has also been found to be effective for the treatment of small-sized vessels [7, 16, 17]. High energies, capable of penetrating the reticular dermis can randomly coagulate dermal blood vessels (random hit theory). FP therefore acts by non-selective photocoagulation and not by a selective effect on blood vessels like selective photothermolysis.

Elimination of epidermal and dermal pigments by the MEND shuttle can be well controlled by adjusting the MTZ density(fill factor). Since the basic principle of nFP does not depend on the properties of the melanin chromophore, all types of skin can be treated by nFP. NFP can therefore be used as valuable alternative for pigmentary problels in patients with darker skin types. Furthermore can nFP be considered even the technique of choice when pigmentation contrast in between the lesion and the surrounding skin are weak as it is often the case in early-stage or moderate photo-aging.

During the last decade, several nFP technologies have been developed using different wavelengths, the according penetration depths; variable pulse durations and operating procedures. For example, a 1,927 nm thulium laser for nFP has been approved by the FDA recently for the treatment of actinic keratosis one of the most common marker of skin- and photo-aging particularly on the face.

Another nFP device uses a Nd:YAG laser emitting at 1,440 and 1,320 nm. The depth of penetration of the 1,440 nm laser is estimated to be 300 µm, whereas the 1,320 nm laser is supposed to be reaching tissue depths of about 500 µm. The device allows sequential emission of the 2 wavelengths from the same fiber with an interval of 15 ms between the pulses. Energy is delivered through a diffractive optic lens assuring the miniaturisation and the production of an MTZ diameter of 100 µm. Using this technique each MTZ is separated by approximately 200 to 500 µm of healthy tissue. According to the device manufacturer the use of a topical anaesthetic cream is not necessary since the forced air cooling used concomitantly with the treament, has an sufficient analgesic effect. Geraghty [18] compared the efficacy of multi-wavelength fractional laser (1,320/1,440 nm) with single wavelength fractional laser (1,440 nm) and assessed the results at 1, 3 and 6 months. Improvements were noted in the studied parameters in all subjects, i.e. texture, dyspigmentation, wrinkles and overall appearance, and no significant differences were observed between the two techniques, although improvement of skin tension was better with the 1,320 nm laser. No side effects were reported Tab. 1. However, these results were recently questioned by Babilas [19] who studied the device for facial skin rejuvenation in 20 patients with moderate photo-aging. The authors found almost no clinical improvement compared to baseline.

Table 1 Brand Device Laser Wavelengths [nm] Delivery method Spot size [mm/MTZ] Energy [mJ/MTZ] Pulse duration [ms]

Brand	Device	Laser	Wave-lengths [nm]	Delivery method	Spot size [mm/MTZ]	Energy [mJ/MTZ]	Pulse duration [ms]
Cynosure	Affirm	Nd:YAG	1320/1440	Stamping	100-150	Up to 4.1	1, 1.5, 2
Lutronic	Mosaic	Er:Glass	1550	Scanned Stamping		4-40	0.5-4.5
Palomar	Lux1540	Er:Glass	1540	Stamping		Up to 100	5, 10
Quanta	Matisse	Er:Glass	1540	Stamping		Up to 20	4-14
Sellas	1550	Er:Glass	1550	Scanned Stamping	312-1000	1-30	0,5
Solta	Faxel re:fine	Er:Glass	1410	Rolling		5-20	
Solta	Fraxel re:store DUAL	Er:Glass	1550/1927	Rolling	135/up to 600	4-70, 5-20	0.015-3

Another 1,540 nm laser device using a handpiece of 10 mm (100 MTZ/cm^2) or of 15 mm (320 mb/cm^2) and an pulse duration of 15 ms has also been introduced. Curiously, the laser was assessed for the treatment of atrophic acne scars and burns but there are no publications on non-ablative facial skin resurfacing [20]. Other lenses allowing more rapid treatment, better cooling and compression enabling deeper dermal penetration have recently been studied only to assess their safety [21]. Another 1,540 nm erbium glass laser was also assessed experimentally, notably combined with PRP for skin rejuvenation [22].

SIDE EFFECTS AND COMPLICATIONS

In a recent retrospective study [23] of 961 treatments, acne-like eruptions were reported in 1.87% of cases in two weeks following the procedure. Furthermore transient, post-inflammatory pigmentation disorders were reported whereas the frequency increased with skin type and energy/MTZ used.

In the follow-up of a cohort of 1,000 fractional photothermolysis treatments, Setyadi [24] evaluated the risk of infectious complications to be 0.2%. The main complication was labial herpes, which can be prevented by the prophylactic administration of antiviral treatment. One case of impetigo was also observed underlining the importance of risk management and following patients up in the post-operative period. Finally, no definitive scars or residual permanent pigment disorders have been published in the framework of skin rejuvenation.

CONCLUSION

The demand for facial skin rejuvenation procedures is on the rise, but patients are demanding procedures to be effective with few post-operative consequences and without the risk of complications.

The effectiveness of NFP is based on a thermally induced neocollagenesis. Its unique thermal damage pattern allows the practitioner to choose from a vast array of possible parameters to generate a personalised response ultimately optimizing the clinical efficacy as well as personalizing post-operative side effects and risks. During the last decade the nFP is hence answering the patients demand for a clinically effective procedure with well adjustable side effects and a very limited number of possible complications.

REFERENCES

[1] Waldorf HA, Kauvar AN, Geronemus RG. Skin resurfacing of fine to deep rhytides using a char free carbon dioxide laser in 47 patients. Dermatol Surg 1995; 21(11): 940-946.

[2] Dover JS, Hruza GJ. Laser skin resurfacing. [Review] Semin Cutan Med Surg 1996; 15(3): 177-188.

[3] Bernstein LJ, Kauvar AN, Grossman MC, Geronemus RG. The short- and long-term side effects of carbon dioxide laser resurfacing. Dermatol Surg 1997; 23(7): 519-525.

[4] Reynolds N, Thomas K, Baker L, Adams C, Kenealy J. Pulsed dye laser and non-ablative wrinkle reduction. Lasers Surg Med 2004; 34(2): 109-113.

[5] Goldberg DJ. New collagen formation after dermal remodeling with an intense pulsed light source. J Cutan Laser Ther 2000; 2(2): 59-61.

[6] Manstein D, Herron GS, Sink RK, Tanner H, Anderson RR. Fractional photothermolysis: a new concept for cutaneous remodeling using microscopic patterns of thermal injury. Lasers Surg Med 2004; 34(5): 426-438.

[7] Laubach HJ, Tannous Z, Anderson RR, Manstein D. Skin responses to fractional photothermolysis. Lasers Surg Med 2006; 38(2): 142-149.
[8] Hantash BM, Bedi VP, Sudireddy V, Struck SK, Herron GS, Chan KF. Laser-induced transepidermal elimination of dermal content by fractional photothermolysis. J Biomed Opt 2006; 11(4): 041115.
[9] Laubach HJ, Manstein D. Fractional photothermolysis. Hautarzt 2007; 58(3): 216-218, 220-223.
[10] Tierney EP, Kouba DJ, Hanke CW. Review of fractional photothermolysis: treatment indications and efficacy. Dermatol Surg 2009; 35: 1445-1461.
[11] Sherling M, Friedman PM, Adrian R, *et al.* Consensus recommandations on the use of an erbium-dopped 1,550 nm fractional laser and its application in dermatologic laser surgery. Dermatol Surg 2010; 36: 461-469.
[12] Fischer GH, Geronemus RG. Short term side effects of fractional photothermolysis. Dermatol Surg 2005; 31(9): 1245-1249.
[13] Tanzi EL, Wanitphakdeedecha R, Alster TS. Fraxel laser indications and long-term follow-up. Aesthet Surg J 2008; 28(6): 675-678; discussion 679-680.
[14] Buis J, Mazer JM. Fractional photo-thermolysis by laser Fraxel as an adjuvant for facial surgical rejuvenation. Ann Chir Plast Esthet 2007; 52(3): 222-233.
[15] Peukert N, Bayer J, Becke D, Zurakowski D, Luger T, Manstein D, Laubach HJ. Fractional photothermolysis for the treatment of facial wrinkles – searching for optimal treatment parameters in a randomized study in the splitface design. J Dtsch Dermatol Ges 2012; 10(12): 898-904.
[16] Behroozan DS, Goldberg LH, Glaich AS, Dai T, Friedman PM. Fractional photothermolysis for treatment of poikiloderma of civatte. Dermatol Surg 2006; 32(2): 298-301.
[17] Glaich AS, Goldberg LH, Dai T, Friedman PM. Fractional photothermolysis for the treatment of telangiectatic matting: a case report. J Cosmet Laser Ther 2007; 9(2): 101-103.
[18] Geraghty LN, Biesman B. Clinical evaluation of a single wavelength fractional laser and a novel multiwavelength fractional laser in the treatment of damaged skin. Laser Surg Med 2009; 41(6): 408-416.
[19] Babilas P, Schreml S, Cames T, Hohenleutner U, Landthaler M, Hohenleutner S. Experience with non ablative fractional phototermolysis with a dual mode device 1,440/1,320 nm: no considerable effect on hypotrophic/acne scars and Facial wrinkles. Laser Med Sci 2011; 26(4): 413-149.
[20] Moravvej H. Barikbin B, Ghavam SA, Karimi S. Non Ablative fractional laser resurfacing. J Laser Med Sci 2011; 2(1): 30-35.
[21] Zelikson B, Walgrave S, *et al.* Evaluation of a fractional laser with optical compression pins. Laser Surg Med 2011; 43: 137-142.
[22] Shin MK, Lee JH, Lee SJ Kim NI. Platelet-rich plasma combined with fractional laser therapyfor skin rejuvenation. Dermatol Surg 2012; 38(4): 623-630.
[23] Graber EM, Tanzi EL, Alster TS. Side effects and complications of fractional laser photothermolysis: an experience with 961 treatments. Dermatol Surg 2008; 34: 301-305.
[24] Setyadi HG, A.A Jacobs, RF Markus. Infectious complications following non ablative fractional resurfacing treatment. Dermatol Surg 2008; 34: 1595-1597.

CHAPTER 7

Ablative fractional laser therapy

Terry Taraneh Farsani, Arisa Ortiz, Mathew Avram

INTRODUCTION

Years of ultraviolet (UV) light exposure induce, among other things, uneven skin tone, roughened skin texture, telangiectasias, rhytides, and decreased skin laxity. Fully ablative carbon dioxide (CO_2) laser and erbium:yttrium-aluminum-garnet (Er:YAG) have been considered the gold standard in skin resurfacing. Although results showed significant clinical improvement in photodamage and tissue laxity, traditional CO_2 laser treatment eventually fell out of favor due to the high risk of treatment complications. These complications include persistent erythema, permanent hypopigmentation, scarring and infection [1, 2]. This led to the development of newer, less aggressive technologies, which have gained popularity due to their safer side effect profiles and decreased postoperative recovery time.

Anderson and Parrish first introduced the concept of selective photothermolysis in 1983 [3]. Selective photothermolysis allows the operator to selectively target light-absorbing molecules, known as chromophores, in the skin by using specific wavelengths of light and appropriate pulse durations. The skin has multiple chromophores including water, hemoglobin, and melanin. Ablative lasers primarily target water. Fractional photothermolysis was first introduced by Manstein *et al.* [4] to address the disadvantages of traditional ablative devices. In fractional photothermolysis, only a fraction of the epidermal and dermal components are treated by delivery of energy into spatially confined microscopic columns, known as microthermal zones (MTZs). These zones comprise approximately 5-70% of the treated skin area per treatment session depending on the treatment density chosen. The first fractionated device was a 1,550 nm nonablative laser system [4]. Although the development of nonablative laser resurfacing has led to safer outcomes, the results are less impressive compared to ablative devices. While nonablative devices induce thermal injury, ablative devices cause vaporization of columns of tissue. Fractional ablative devices induce areas of vaporization with surrounding coagulative necrosis and transepidermal elimination of the necrotic debris within 7-10 days. This process stimulates new collagen formation.

Since there is sparing of intact follicular units, stem cells and fibroblasts surrounding each MTZ, this results in faster re-epithelialization, tissue contraction, and stimulation of collagen [4]. In contrast, fully ablative laser therapy results in complete removal of the entire epidermis as well as a portion of the dermis, requiring increased recovery time, increased risk of infection, and increased risk of scarring and delayed hypopigmentation.

Skin resurfacing using fractional photothermolysis can produce clinical results approaching those of traditional ablative, with decreased recovery time and improved safety profile, when compared to fully ablative laser resurfacing.

TECHNICAL ASPECTS

Ablative fractional lasers include fractional CO_2, erbium:yttrium-aluminum-garnet (Er:YAG) and YSGG lasers (2,970-nm). CO_2 lasers emit light at a wavelength of 10,600-nm, targeting water as its chromophore. The Er:YAG laser emits light at a wavelength of 2,940-nm and also targets water, though more precisely given water has the same absorption peak. When fractionated, these lasers use a lens and adjustable beam to focus the energy within the dermis, creating deep ablative columns, but limiting thermal damage to specific areas. These MTZs span from the epidermis down to the reticular dermis. These are the first laser devices to achieve this safely, compared to traditional ablative devices, which can only achieve thermal ablation down to the papillary dermis without inducing scarring. The CO_2 lasers may penetrate to a depth of 1.6 mm. The Er:Yag ablative fractional device produces micro holes with diameter of 50-150 microns, penetrates to a depth of 0.1-1 mm, and produces a coagulation zone between 5-50 microns. Pulse width determines thickness of the coagulation zone, which increases with increasing pulse width. Although fractionation decreases the risk of scarring, greater density of MTZs, higher energy or fluence, and a higher number of passes increase the risk of bulk dermal heating, epidermal injury, and consequently, treatment-related adverse effects and downtime [5-7].

There are currently several devices that use fractional resurfacing technology. These devices use either a scanning or stamping mechanism to deliver fractional energy. The energy settings determine the depth of penetration, while the density determines the percent coverage. Fractional technologies can never achieve 100% coverage, but can approach traditional ablative coverage by increasing the number of passes. Caution needs to be employed as higher densities greatly increase the risk for hypertrophic scarring.

Ablative fractional CO_2 lasers include FraxelRe:pair (SoltaMedical, Hayward, CA), Pixel Perfect (Alma Lasers, Buffalo Grove, IL), the Smartxide DOT (DEKA Medical Inc, San Francisco, CA), Ellipse Juvia (Del Mar Technologies, San Marcos, CA), MixtoSX (LASERINGusa, San Ramon, CA), Active and Deep and Total FX with UltraPulse (Lumenis, San Jose, CA) and eCO_2 (Lutronic, Fremont, CA). Erbium-YAG types include the Pixel XL (Alma Lasers, Buffalo Grove, IL), Lux2940 (Palomar Medical Technologies Inc, Burlington, MA), and PROfractionalTherapy (Sciton, Palo Alto, CA) Tab. 1.

The FraxelRe;pair uses a scanning mechanism of action and allows for treatment energies up to 70 mJ/cm^2. ActiveFX utilizes a computerized pattern generator with a 1.3 mm spot size for photo damage. It may be used in the CoolScan mode, allowing for non-linear scanning to increase patient comfort. DeepFX also uses computerized pattern generator in conjunction with the UltraPulse Encore to deliver 0.1 mm spot size in a fractional mode covering a treated surface area up to 25% greater than other fractional technologies, resulting in more effective tightening of deep rhytides. The depth of ablation, and resulting thermal damage, depends on energy density and the number of stacked pulses (maximum 5). TotalFX combines use of DeepFX, followed by ActiveFX for maximum effect. It is important to note that manufacturers calculate densities differently, with some only including the zone of ablation while others include the zone of ablation as well as the surrounding area of coagulative necrosis as well. Thus, confusion between densities among various devices can lead to complications.

Table 1

Manufacturer	Wavelength (nm)	Pulse duration (milliseconds)	Delivery	Spot size (um)	Scanner size (mm)	Depth (um)
FraxelRe:pair (Solta Medical)	10,600 CO_2	0.15-3	IOTS (continuous motion)	< 140	n/a	1,600
Pixel Perfect (Alma Lasers)	10,600 CO_2	0.05-0.1	Super Pulse	150	7 × 7 and 9 × 9	25-300
Smartxide DOT (DEKA Medical Inc)	10,600 CO_2	200 microseconds or 2 ms	Scanned	350	15 × 15	200-1,500
Ellipse Juvia (Del Mar Technologies	10,600 CO_2	2-7	Scanned	500	7 × 7 × 9 × 11	400
Mixto SX (Lasering USA)	10,600 CO_2	2.5-16	Scanned	300/180	20 × 20	Ablation: 200 Thermal damage: 300
Active, Deep, and Total FX with Ultraplus (Lumenis)	10,600 CO_2	< 1	Scanned	1,300/120	9 × 9/10 × 10	10-300 (1,300 spot), 150-1,600 (120), up to 3,200 with pulse stack
eCO_2 (Lutronic)	10,600 CO_2	Changes with energy setting	Stamping	1,000/300/120	14 × 14	2,500
Pixel XL (Alma Lasers)	2940 Er:YAG	1, 1.5, or 2	Scanned	250	11 × 11	20-50
Lux 2940 (Palomar Medical Technologies Inc)	2940 Er:YAG	0.2-0.5	Stamping	100	10 × 10/6 × 6	200
PROfractionalTherapy (Sciton)	2940 Er:YAG	Changes with energy setting	Scanned	430/250	20 × 20	1,500

INDICATIONS

Although this chapter focuses on photoaging, fractional photothermolysis has been used for many applications including redundant skin resulting from involution of hemangiomas, acne scarring [8], and surgical, burn and traumatic scars. In general, fine and moderate facial rhytides, solar elastosis, laxity, vascular dyschromia and lentigines have been successfully treated with fractional ablative resurfacing [9]. Another application for ablative fractional photothermolysis is laser-assisted transdermal drug delivery [10].

PATIENT SELECTION

Selecting the proper patient is critical to obtaining optimal results. During the consultation visit, examination of the proposed treatment area should be performed. Sun exposure prior to and possible sun exposure after the procedure may increase risk of post-treatment skin hyperpigmentation and must be avoided. History of keloid or hypertrophic scar formation increases risk of these complications post-procedure. Skin phototype should be noted, as Fitzpatrick skin types I-II experience less risk of postoperative hyperpigmentation than darker skin phototypes. While any skin type may be treated with fractional ablative lasers, skin types V-VI should be approached with caution and should be treated at low-density setting to decrease the risk for pigmentary complications. In addition, any suspicious pigmented lesions should be biopsied for histologic examination prior to laser treatment.

A thorough history should be performed. Prior procedures, including dermabrasion, cryosurgery, and deep chemical peels, may have resulted in underlying fibrosis or pigment alteration. History of blepharoplasty increases risk for ectropion formation. A way to test for patients who may be more susceptible to this potential complication would include performing a “snap test”. Lower lid laxity with slow retraction when the lid is pulled down and released, would indicate increased likelihood of ectropion [11]. Fractional ablative laser therapy may unmask these unwanted findings. History of labial herpes may result in reactivation or dissemination of the virus following laser therapy. If the virus reactivates and is not diagnosed and treated rapidly, there is a risk of scarring; therefore it is imperative that all patients receive antiviral prophylaxis beginning one day prior to the procedure [12]. Other infections, such as warts, may spread after treatment [13, 14]. Skin disorders known to exhibit koebnerization, such as lichen planus, vitiligo, and psoriasis have the potential to worsen. Autoimmune disorders may result in decreased immunologic function and collagen repair mechanisms, decreasing the ability of the tissue to heal well. Medication history should include prior treatment with isotretinoin, which delays wound healing and collagen formation, and may result in hypertrophic scarring. Most practitioners wait 6-12 months after cessation of oral retinoid treatment prior to treating the patient. Smoking should cease prior to and after treatment as smoking can impede the wound healing process. Patients with acne should be treated for their acne with the appropriate topical or systemic antibiotics prior to laser treatment, as use of occlusive ointments in the postoperative period may worsen acne, complicating the postoperative course.

Lastly, setting realistic expectations is integral to patient satisfaction. Overall cosmetic outcome from a single treatment are best realized at 3 to 6 months following treatment, as collagen remodeling continues up to 6 months [15]. Most patients receive one to two treatments, but those with more moderate to severe photodamage may require more. Patients with unrealistic expectations are not favorable candidates. In addition, treatment should be limited to those who are physically and emotionally able to handle the expected postoperative course and instructions.

PREOPERATIVE MANAGEMENT

All patients, regardless of whether they have history of herpes labialis, should start prophylactic antiviral medication 1 day prior to treatment and continue for at least 7 days. Prophylaxis with oral antibiotics may also be prescribed to reduce the risk of bacterial infection. Our practice uses valacyclovir 500 mg twice daily and dicloxacillin 500 mg twice daily beginning 24 hours prior to the procedure. Drug allergy needs to be assessed prior to prescribing medications. Pain control is managed with a topical anesthetic (EMLA, LMX) and is applied while the patient is in the office 60 minutes prior to the procedure. In our practice, 23% lidocaine combined with 7% tetracaine is used 1 hour prior to the procedure. Caution must be taken in applying high strength topical anesthetics over a large area given potential cardiac adverse effects. Despite anesthetic application, the treatment can still be quite painful. Supplemental nerve blocks, including the supraorbital, infraorbital, nasalis, and mental nerve blocks, may also be administered for greater anesthetic coverage 15 minutes prior to the procedure using lidocaine 1% to 2% with 1:100,000 or 1:200,000 epinephrine. Local infiltration of lidocaine to areas that are not anesthetized with nerve blocks, such as the lateral parts of the face, may be performed. Topical anesthetic cream is removed prior to the procedure. In addition, intramuscular non-steroidal anti-inflammatory medications may be given for additional pain control. Anti-anxiolytics may be used to help calm an anxious patient. In some cases, general anesthesia may be used with an anesthesiologist present. However, one must ensure a family member or friend is present to accompany and transport the patient home after the treatment has been completed. Severe pain post-operatively is very rare. The best explanation is that the heat generated by the treatment is released through the ablative channels during and after the procedure. More commonly, minor pain is described as a mild sunburn for the first 24 hours. More significant pain may be a sign of complication and merits further exploration.

CLINICAL STUDIES

The first clinical investigation evaluating fractional deep dermal ablation for photodamaged skin demonstrated that fractional CO_2 laser was an effective modality for resurfacing with an improved safety profile compared to traditional resurfacing [16]. Subjects received 1-2 treatment on the face and neck with fluences ranging from 10 to 40 mJ/MTZ and densities ranging from 400 to 1,200 MTZ/cm [10]. Eighty-three percent of subjects achieved 50-100% overall improvement based on a quartile scale assessing improvement in rhytides, pigmentation, texture, laxity and overall appearance 1 and 3 months post-treatment. Treatments were well tolerated without any serious adverse events. These results compare favorably to non-ablative fractional technologies.

A small study comparing four sessions of fractional versus one session of ablative (Er:YAG) laser resurfacing for facial rejuvenation, revealed similar objective benefits [17]. Six patients were included in each arm of the study. Biopsy specimens were obtained prior to laser resurfacing treatment and at 1 and 6 months. Histologically, both treatments resulted in increased epidermal thickness, neocollagen with increased collagen types I, III, and VII, as well as tropoelastin formation. However, epidermal thickness, elastin, and tropoelastin concentrations were more marked in the ablative laser group.

A prospective study of 45 patients with moderate to severe photoaging reported their 6-month post-treatment clinical results after receiving two to three ablative fractional laser treatments at 8-week intervals [18]. Clinical measurement was performed by a blinded physician via clinical photographic assessment, using a modified photoaging scale. Results revealed a mean improvement of 48.5% for skin texture, 50.3% for skin laxity, 53.9% for dyschromia, and 52.4% for overall cosmetic outcome (all $p < 0.05$) Fig. 1.

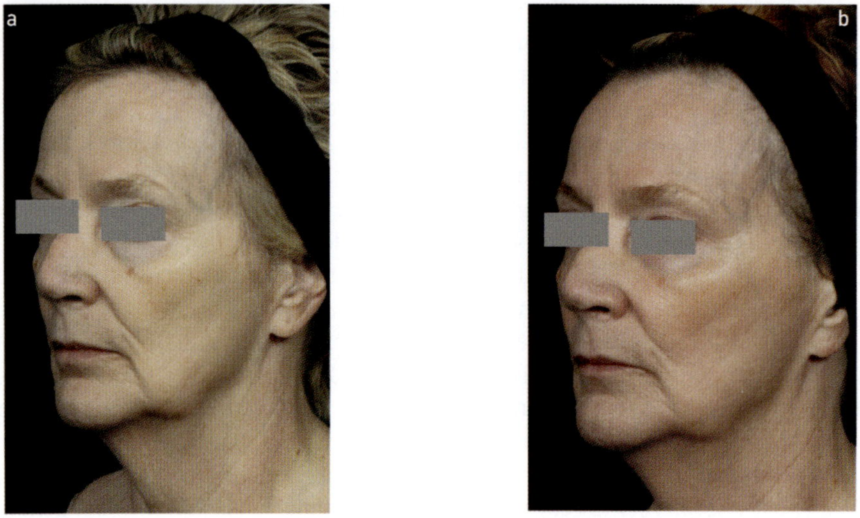

Figure 1 Fractionated ablative laser before treatment (a), results 3 months later (b)

A more recent prospective study for the treatment of photoaging was performed in 10 patients. Assessment of laser efficacy was determined by two methods: histologic examination reporting the correlation between pulse duration and ablation depth, as well as blinded physician clinical photographic assessment [19]. Patients were randomized to one of four pulse duration settings (500, 1,000, 1,500, and 1,800 µs). Results showed improvement in all clinical categories at 6-months post-treatment. This included 47.5% improvement in dyschromia, 56% in skin texture and in skin laxity, 52.5% in rhytides, and 61.5% improvement in overall cosmetic outcome. Histopathology revealed a proportional increase in thermal coagulation depth with increase in pulse duration. Pulse duration of 1,800 µs correlated with an ablation depth of 1.1 mm, which targets the reticular dermis and was shown to be safe.

With the advent of new fractional photothermolysis technologies, patients now experience significant clinical improvement in rhytides and photodamage, with less post-operative recovery time than with ablative treatments. Complete re-epithelialization generally occurs within 3-6 days, resulting in fewer infections, less risk of acneiform eruptions associated with use of occlusive ointments, less erythema and swelling, and decreased risk of scarring with hyper- or hypopigmentation [20]. Campbell *et al.* performed a retrospective evaluation of 373 treatments, without evidence of scarring [21]. In a recent retrospective review of 490 treatments in 374 patients, there were no reports of scarring or hypopigmentation [22]. These results are consistent with the improved safety profile of fractional ablative devices. Nonetheless, it is important to note that there is a clear risk of scarring, especially at higher treatment densities, particularly on the neck [5-7]. Caution should be exercised with these devices. It is imperative that the laser surgeon is able to recognize and treat complications that may occur.

Long-term efficacy of fractional ablative devices for photoaging has shown 67% maintenance of improvement at 2 years when compared to improvement seen at 3-month follow-up [22]. While subjects seem to maintain improvement on the long-term, there is some relaxation of the initial tightening. The authors speculate that some of the initial improvement observed is enhanced by persistent inflammation and collagen remodeling. The natural progression of aging also contributes to the decrease in improvement over time. Therefore, patients will likely need touch-up treatments every few years to maintain improvement.

COMBINATION TREATMENTS

Ablative fractional treatments may be combined with non-ablative fractional laser treatments. For instance, ablative fractional treatment may be used on the eyelids and upper lip rhytides, whereas non-ablative treatment is performed on the cheeks and forehead.

Other combination treatments may include ablative fractional laser treatment with superficial laser peels targeting the mid to deep epidermal surface. The laser peel targets superficial photodamage while fractional ablative laser therapy targets deeper rhytides, decreasing perioral and periorbital rhytides.

PRACTICAL TIPS

Technique is highly variable, and is physician- and device-dependent. Laser surgeons should understand the extent of tissue injury produced by the specific device used at various settings. Skin thickness should be considered, as eyelid skin will require lower fluences since eyelid skin is thinner than other areas of the face. The neck is a high-risk area for scarring given that the skin is thinner and there is paucity of adnexal structures. This is especially true for patients who have undergone previous surgical lifting procedures. Both lower fluences and lower densities should be used when treating the neck as well as the jawline in patients with a history of lifting procedures. Guides and textbooks are available, demonstrating the thickness of skin and number of adnexal structures at various anatomic sites. These may be helpful in guiding the physician in the choice of appropriate and safe laser settings. Each cosmetic unit is treated separately, with care to minimize bulk heating. Bulk heating is minimized by lowering treatment densities and allowing sufficient time for the skin to cool between passes. This is especially true when a small anatomic area is being treated. During the treatment, a cooling device can be used to help minimize pain. Edema, erythema, oozing, and pinpoint bleeding are typically observed during the procedure and immediately after. Post-operative photos should be shown to a patient prior to treatment to avoid post-treatment surprise as to the extent of these side effects.

POSTOPERATIVE CARE

Immediately after the procedure, cold compresses may be applied to help decrease swelling. The face should be washed with gentle cleanser and water, followed by application of petrolatum ointment or other emollient with gauze soaks. Proper postoperative wound care is integral to optimizing long-term results. The treated area should be kept moist for proper healing and to decrease the risk of scarring, as the presence of crusting or eschar may impede keratinocyte migration and re-epithelialization. Soaks with distilled water or diluted vinegar every few hours for the first 24-48 hours may help decrease crust formation. Many physicians are proponents of frequent application of thick healing ointment to the skin surface, whereas others favor occlusive or semi-occlusive dressings placed on the treated skin. While the latter may increase patient comfort and decrease patient involvement in wound care, this method may also result in additional expenses for the patient and a potentially higher risk of infection. Patients interestingly experience little post-procedure pain, which is thought due to heat released through ablated MTZ channels. Follow-up is recommended at 48-72 hours post-procedure or sooner. Significant pain more than 24 hours after treatment should be monitored.

There have not been any studies assessing whether decreasing the inflammatory response has an effect on efficacy. In addition, cool compresses and anti-inflammatory medications are encouraged. The patient should avoid rubbing or scratching the treated skin, and should not apply topical retinoic acid derivatives, glycolic acid, and fragrance-containing products or cosmetics in the preoperative and postoperative period. Re-epithelialization typically occurs on post-operative day 3, with improvement in erythema and edema. After this has taken place, strict sun avoidance is important to prevent postoperative skin darkening.

REDUCING ADVERSE EFFECTS: EXPECTED SIDE EFFECTS AND POTENTIAL COMPLICATIONS

The main advantage of fractional ablative resurfacing when compared to fully ablative treatments is that the former has a safer side effect profile, while approaching results of traditional ablative devices. Nonetheless, side effects may still occur and are typically related to the expertise of the laser surgeon, the area treated, and the skin phototype of the patient. While edema, erythema, pinpoint bleeding and pruritus are expected in the immediate postoperative period, these are temporary and normally resolve within the first few weeks of healing Fig. 2.

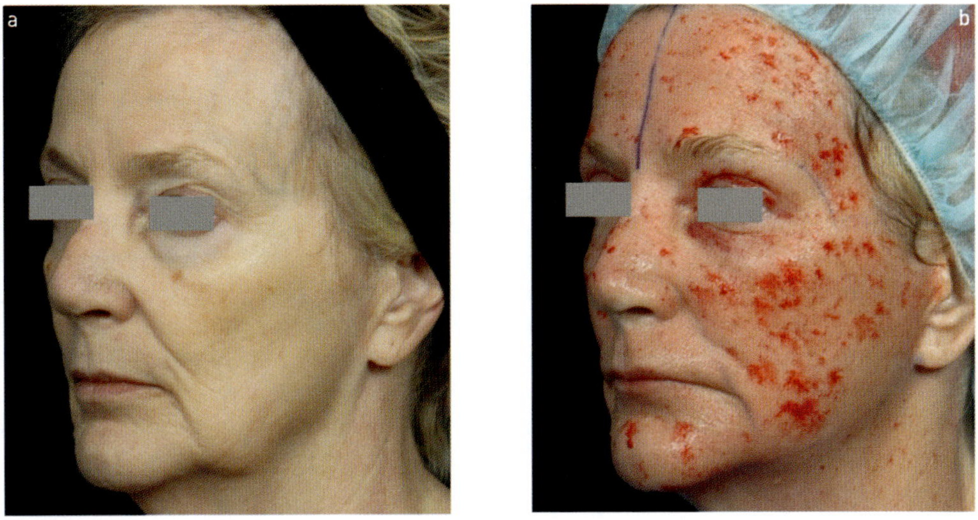

Figure 2 Fractional ablative resurfacing before treatment (a), immediately after treatment (b)

Minor complications include temporary milia formation and acne exacerbation, which may be due to use of occlusive dressings and/or ointments [24]. This risk is increased in those prone to acne, underscoring the importance of treating and controlling acne prior to the procedure. Although milia and acne usually resolve spontaneously over time, oral antibiotics may be prescribed for those with resistant acne flares not responding to topical antibiotics. Risk of contact dermatitis, usually irritant, may occur with use of topical creams, medications, or soap, as there is disruption in skin barrier function following the procedure.

Moderate adverse effects include post-operative bacterial infection with *Staphylococcus, Pseudomonas*, and Klebsiella have been reported [25]. Fungal infection and viral infection may also occur and should be treated aggressively with the proper anti-infective agent. Disseminated herpes simplex infections may require intravenous anti-viral treatment [27]. Herpetic infection may present as erosions without intact vesicles given the denuded lased skin. A clue to infection is increasing pain after the procedure. Any patient with increasing pain should be brought back for immediate evaluation and antimicrobial cultures. Treatment with broad-spectrum antibiotics may be initiated while awaiting culture results. An untreated bacterial infection of the jaw line or earlobe area may result in the development of a life-threatening neck abscess if not treated early [11]. The procedure should only be performed by a physician who can recognize and treat such infections. Transient hyperpigmentation is one of the more common side effects, with an increased risk in darker skinned patients. Pre-treatment with hydroquinone and use of sunscreens may be given to high-risk patients 1 month prior to the procedure to help prevent hyperpigmentation, although data demonstrating efficacy is lacking. A bronze discoloration, thought to be due to transepidermal elimination of necrotic debris containing melanin, may also persist for weeks following treatment. Although this hyperpigmentation is transient, treatment with topical hydroquinone, retinoic, azeleic, and glycolic acid, may be restarted 3 weeks after the procedure to help hasten resolution. Hydroquinone treatment should not last more than 3 months, as the risk of post-treatment hypopigmentation and ochronosis increase with longer periods of treatment.

Granuloma formation following fractional laser therapy has been reported. This resolved with scarring 4 months after treatment with intermittent topical corticosteroid treatment [11].

Severe complications include hypertrophic scarring and ectropion formation. Ten cases of post-ablative fractional CO_2 laser scarring have been reported in the literature to date [5, 7]. Ectropion and lagopthalmus have occurred with treatment of the upper and lower eyelids, and are more common when treating patients with previous blepharoplasty. Significant swelling of the infraorbital area postoperatively should be treated with class I topical corticosteroid ointment to avoid ectropion formation. Ross *et al.* encountered a case of scarring and persistent erythema nine days post treatment [5]. Avram *et al.* [6] report five cases of scarring in patients who were referred to his practice 1-3 month's following ablative fractional laser treatment of the neck region. Two of these cases are discussed in detail and include the treatment parameters that likely resulted in excessive thermal injury via excessive overlap of laser application. The thin skin and decreased pilosebaceous units make the neck more prone to scarring in comparison to facial skin. In the second case discussed by Avram *et al.*, wound infection may have complicated the post-operative course, resulting in an increased risk of hypertrophic scarring.

In general, the neck, chest, and jawline areas are at highest risk for scarring, and aggressive high-energy treatments increase this risk. Further risks for scarring include previous plastic surgical procedures, such as a neck lift, which produce mild fibrosis and alter the cutaneous vasculature and impede normal wound healing after fractional laser therapy. Following a neck lift, the neck skin may be pulled upward and placed on facial sites, resulting in increased risk of scarring in these areas.

This highlights the importance of careful history taking, to avoid treatment of these areas with energies similar to treating facial skin. Fife *et al.* [7] also report scarring in four cases after fractional CO_2 laser therapy to areas such as the neck, eyelids, and chest, with an increased risk of scarring if infection ensues.

SUMMARY

In summary, use of fractional ablative lasers for treatment of mild to moderate rhytides and facial photodamage provides an improved side effect profile and reduced postoperative morbidity in comparison to fully ablative techniques. Additional treatments may be necessary to maintain improvement long-term. Careful patient selection and proper technique and treatment parameters are imperative in obtaining optimal results. Lastly, the importance of postoperative care and follow-up cannot be overemphasized.

REFERENCES

[1] Nanni CA, Alster TS. Complications of carbon dioxide laser resurfacing. An evaluation of 500 patients. Dermatol Surg Mar 1998; 24(3): 315-320.
[2] Alster TS, Nanni CA, Williams CM. Comparison of four carbon dioxide resurfacing lasers. A clinical and histopathologic evaluation. Dermatol Surg Mar 1999; 25(3): 153-158; discussion 159.
[3] Anderson RR, Parrish JA. Selective photothermolysis: precise microsurgery by selective absorption of pulsed radiation. Science 1983; 220: 524-527.
[4] Manstein D, Herron GS, Sink RK, Tanner H, Anderson RR. Fractional photothermolysis: a new concept for cutaneous remodeling using microscopic patterns of thermal injury. Lasers Surg Med 2004; 34(5): 426-438.
[5] Ross, *et al.* Scarring and persistent erythema after fractionated ablative CO_2 laser resurfacing. J Drugs Dermatol 2008; 7(11): 1072-1073.
[6] Avram MM, Tope WD, Yu T, Szachowicz E, Nelson JS. Hypertrophic scarring of the neck following ablative fractional carbon dioxide laser resurfacing. Lasers Surg Med 2009; 41(3): 185-188.
[7] Fife D, *et al.* Complications of fractional CO_2 laser resurfacing: four cases. Lasers Surg Med 2009; 41: 179-184.
[8] Walgrave SE, Ortiz AE, MacFalls HT, Elkeeb L, Truitt AK, Tournas JA, Zelickson BD, Zachary CB. Evaluation of a novel fractional resurfacing device for treatment of acne scarring. Lasers Surg Med 2009 Feb; 41(2): 122-7. doi: 10.1002/lsm.20725.
[9] Tierney EP, Hanke CW. Fractionated carbon dioxide laser treatment of photoaging: Prospective study in 45 patients and review of the literature. Dermatol Surg 2011; 37: 1279-1290.
[10] Waibel JS, Wulkan AJ, Shumaker PR. Treatment of hypertrophic scars using laser and laser assisted corticosteroid delivery. Lasers Surg Med 2013; 45(3): 135-140.
[11] Rendon-Pellerano MI, Lentini J, Eaglstein WE, Kirsner RS, Hanft K, Pardo RJ. Laser resurfacing: usual and unusual complications. Dermatol Surg 1999; 25(5): 360.
[12] Naouri M, Delage M, Khallouf R, Georgesco G, Atlan M. CO_2 fractional resurfacing: side effects and immediate complications. Ann Dermatol Venereol 2011; 138(1): 7-10.
[13] Van der Lei B, van Schijndel AW, Blanken R. Exacerbation of multiple plane warts following laser skin resurfacing. Aesthet Surg J 2006; 26(3): 297-299.
[14] Torezan LA, Osorio N, Neto CF. Development of multiple warts after skin resurfacing with CO_2 laser. Dermatol Surg 2000; 26(1): 70-72.
[15] Alexiades-Armenakas MR, Dover JS, Arndr KA. The spectrum of laser skin resurfacing: Non-ablative, fractional, and ablative laser resurfacing. J Am Acad Dermatol 2008; 58: 719-737.
[16] Rahman Z, MacFalls H, Jiang K, Chan KF, Kelly K, Tournas J, *et al.* Fractional deep dermal ablation induces tissue tightening. Lasers Surg Med 2009; 41(2): 78-86.
[17] El-Domyati, *et al.* Fractional versus ablative erbium-yttrium-aluminum-garnet laser resurfacing for facial rejuvenation: An objective evaluation. J Am Acad Dermatol 2013; 68(1): 103-112.
[18] Tierney EP, Hanke CW. Fractionated carbon dioxide laser treatment of photoaging: Prospective study in 45 patients and review of the literature. Dermatol Surg 2011; 37: 1279-1290.
[19] Tierney EP, Hanke CW, Petersen J. Ablative fractionated CO_2 laser treatment of photoaging: A clinical and histologic study. Dermatol Surg 2012; 38(11): 1177-1189.
[20] Tierney, *et al.* Fractionated CO_2 laser skin rejuvenation. Dermatol Ther 2011; (24): 41-53.
[21] Campbell, *et al.* Adverse events of fractionated carbon dioxide laser: review of 373 treatments. Dermatol Surg 2010; 36(11): 1645-1650.
[22] Shamsaldeen, *et al.* The adverse events of deep fractional CO_2: a retrospective study of 490 treatments in 374 patients. Lasers Surg Med 2011; 43(6): 453-456.
[23] Ortiz AE, Tremaine AM, Zachary CB. Long-term efficacy of a fractional resurfacing device. Lasers Surg Med Feb 2010; 42(2): 168-170.
[24] Sullivan SA, Dailey RA. Complications of laser resurfacing and their management. Opthal Plast Reconstr Surg 2000; 16(6): 417-426.

[25] Ortiz AE, Tingey C, Yu YE, Ross EV. Topical steroids implicated in postoperative infection following ablative laser resurfacing. Lasers Surg Med Jan 2012; 44(1): 1-3.
[26] Sriprachya-anunt S, *et al.* Infections complicating pulsed carbon dioxide laser resurfacing for photoaged facial skin. Dermatol Surg 1997; 23: 527-536.
[27] Fitzpatrick RE, Goldman MP, Sature NM, *et al.* Pulsed carbon dioxide laser resurfacing of photoaged skin. Arch Dermatol 1996; 132: 395-402.

CHAPTER 8

Fractional radiofrequency

Klaus Fritz, George Sorin Tiplica

RADIOFREQUENCIES

The electromagnetic energy of radio frequencies (300 MHz-3 KHz) produces an electrical current that has the property to generate heat which flows through the resistance of the dermis and the hypodermis.

The energy is transferred from the electric field to the charged particles of the targeted tissue through the electrons and ions. The heat is produced as a result of the movement of particles within the electric field. This resistance is called impedance and it generates heat when the electrical current is converted into thermal energy. The quantity of the energy being produced can be defined by the following formula:

Energy (J) = I2 × z × t

I: current; z: impedance; t: time in seconds

Electrical conductivity affects the penetration depth of the radiofrequency energy. The penetration depth of this energy, expressed in millimeters, is inversely proportional to the square root of the frequency. The lower the frequencies, the higher the penetration rates are. It is necessary to be able to control the depth of the heating of this type of system which is designed to treat the body and facial areas. Electric fields resulting from radio waves can further heat deeper tissues, such as the dermis and fatty tissues, than the skin or the muscles. This method is frequently used to treat skin sagging, cellulitis, wrinkles or acne scars, as well as to remodel the face and the body. Certain new devices are able to reach the deepest fat layers and to reduce body fat.

Radiofrequency energy is a form of electromagnetic energy (300 MHz-3 KHz) that produces an electrical current, which generates heat as a result of tissue resistance [1, 2].

In contrast to most lasers, which target specific chromophores, RF depends on electrical properties of target tissue and is chromophore-independent, and thus is expected to have better safety profiles for all skin types [3].

There are different types of RF for medical use:

– unipolar: using a single electrode. Most of the energy is deposited at the boundaries of the electrode, therefore intensive cooling is required to protect the epidermis, and higher powers are needed for substantial heating of deep layers;

– bipolar: the electrical current flows between two electrodes at a fixed distance. The penetration depth equals half of the distance between the electrodes, so it is very limited in penetration depth. It usually does not go beyond the epidermis, if delivered at the skin and not in the skin;

– multisource phase-controlled: the devices use multiple independent RF sources, controlled by a microprocessor. The multisource RF technology (3DEEP by Endymed Medical, Cesarea, Israel) uses the repulsion between the electromagnetic fields with different phases to enhance depth of penetration of energy while minimizing energy flow on the skin surface [4].

The heat which is produced as a result of radiofrequencies stimulates certain fibroblasts, which leads to the denaturation of the collagen. The heated fibroblasts contribute to the remodeling of the tissues.

In order to be effective, temperatures have to range between 39° C and 42° C for more than 5 minutes. It is possible to get better results by applying higher levels of heat, which can even lead to the contraction of the tissues. It then becomes more difficult to balance the effects of the treatment, as well as the side-effects. Regarding skin tightening, application temperatures are frequently higher (for instance, with Thermage, Solta Medical, Inc, Hayward, California equipment). Regarding remodeling, the necessary heat quantity is minimal, but the application must last 5 to 15 minutes for each treated area, and requires multiple sessions in order to obtain the stimulation effect.

Studies show that 1 to 4 months are required for the improvement of facial skin sagging. Results gained with the radiofrequency treatment are mild to moderate, but the treatment is well tolerated, has few side-effects and does not require absence from work, or very little.

Radiofrequency technology is not always sufficient on its own in order to raise the tissue temperature at these levels. Particularly, in its bipolar version, the treatment is limited to a rather superficial penetration and has to be combined with other technologies. Some equipment initially proceed with the pre-heating of the tissues by infrared, which modifies impedance and allows radiofrequencies to penetrate in more depth (Velashape/ELOS technology). This equipment uses superficial cooling not only to protect the main area of contact, but especially to apply sufficient amounts of heat, which are then transmitted through the cooled superficial layers to the non cooled deep layers. This cooling system provides deeper radiofrequency penetration. Some manufacturers use ultrasound (Exilis BTL), pulsed magnetic fields (Venus Freeze) or vacuum (Viora/Syneron) in order to submit the tissue to aspiration, to thin the epidermis and to diffuse radiofrequencies, not from above, but laterally, which allows to reach deeper layers.

Through these modified technologies, radiofrequency is the most commonly used method of body remodeling and allows the use of non-invasive treatments aimed at skin tightening, fat reduction and smoothening.

FRACTIONAL RF

The currently available treatments for depressed scars and rejuvenation include ablative and non-ablative laser treatments, full and fractional, chemical peels of light to deep types, and micro-needling. Ablative lasers – also in fractional mode – cannot avoid downtime. Most existing fractional laser devices are either too aggressive and are associated with high level of patient discomfort, downtime and high adverse effect rate, or they lack the ability to generate full volumetric heating for collagen remodeling.

Radiofrequency plays an increasing role in heating the dermis and ablating the epidermis with less downtime.

Fractional RF treatments are mainly used to enhance the skin texture, to reduce the skin sagging, to remedy dilated pores and scars, as well as to rejuvenate.

Technologies

RF is delivered within the skin layers, in spite of being applied to the skin surface. Radiofrequency is fractionated, leading to the effraction of the epidermis, which can be compared to other fractional systems.

Furthermore, there are fractional RF devices that include micro-needles, which penetrate the epidermis without resulting in skin lesions, in order to deliver energy in the dermal layer.

There is no epidermal damage, nor is there any epidermal effect irrespective of how high the applied fluence. Heat can be delivered to the dermis without ablation or downtime if the epidermis is not ablated. Such systems are available for bipolar and unipolar RF.

In body contouring, numerous RF devices are available to heat up the deep tissue. Fractional RF devices are minimally invasive systems that deliver RF current through an array of electrodes to pinpoint the source of symptoms in the areas to be treated – leaving surrounding tissue unharmed. Treating a "fraction" of the skin with a laser or RF creates islands of treated skin in a sea of untreated skin. The benefits of the fractional approach are reduced wound healing time and reduced complications.

Fractional RF treatments can induce neoelastogenesis and neocollagenesis initiated by a wound healing response. Optimal skin remodeling requires thermal effect on both epidermis and dermis. An optimal solution will combine three types of effects: minimal ablation on the surface for textural improvement, controlled dermal coagulation for tissue renewal and overall volumetric heating for collagen stimulation.

Selection of available devices

Currently, there is a limited number of devices and technologies available for fractional radiofrequency.

E-Matrix/E-Two (Syneron)

It uses the Matrix RF (Syneron) hand-held applicator, a bipolar RF-based device delivering RF energy that is tunable for ablation, coagulation and heating.

The tip consists of parallel rows of bipolar-arranged gold-covered electrode pins, per 82 × 12 mm that form an array of positively and negatively charged electrodes, delivering bipolar RF energy in a fractional manner. An energy level limit of 20 J can be delivered at either 5 or 10% coverage rate via 64 equally spaced electrode pins; each pin has a diameter of ~ 200 microns. The fractional resurfacing using this RF device has been termed "sublative rejuvenation" because the skin remodeling occurs deep below the epidermal surface and at sublative levels of heating [5].

The treatment parameters are determined based on the severity of the preexisting skin conditions, distribution of lesions, specific anatomical location, and proximity of bones and consisted of three programs:

- A (coverage rate 5%, 10%; presets 4-8 J);
- B (coverage rate 5%, 10%; presets 8-16 J);
- C (coverage rate 5%, 10%; presets 17-25 J).

Treatment is delivered in a single, non-overlapping pass over the treatment area. The preferred irradiation end point is mild erythema on the treated area.

EndyMed

It is an FDA-cleared computerized multiple phase controlled RF generator, that generates pulses of RF energy, which are emitted into the skin, causing a non-ablative deep dermal heating effect, resulting in skin tightening. The FSR handpiece contains a matrix of 112 micro-ablative dots (tiny RF electrodes), allowing simultaneous fractional micro-ablation of the epidermis together with volumetric heating of 100% of the dermis. The system uses microprocessor controlled 6 independent RF sources, that provide the ability to differentiate between micro-ablation and dermal heating.

The major advantage of the multisource fractional skin resurfacing technology used by Endymed is that in addition to its fractional skin ablation of the epidermis, it allows volumetric heating up to 2.8 mm. The use of multiple RF sources allows in addition homogenous fractional skin ablation with minimized pain [6] Fig. 1.

V-touch System

SVC™ technology (Viora V-touch) stands for the combination of Switching, Vacuum and Cooling mechanisms, which is designed to enhance clinical results, patients' safety and comfort.

Switching technology makes it possible to reduce skin impedance before the fractional pulse and selectively chooses depth penetration of the RF current, creating volumetric heating of the target area before releasing the fractional pulse. Since the tissue conductivity of RF energy is significantly correlated to tissue temperature, an increase in skin temperature lowers skin impedance. Consequently, the target tissue is selectively heated by the RF current [2].

Pre-heating of the target tissue increases skin conductivity prior to the fractional pulse and reduces the energy levels needed, reducing patients' pain levels and post-operative complications. The vacuum-induced skin flattening creates pressure on the nerves of the skin, which leads to significant pain reduction. Cooling: if the temperature of the target

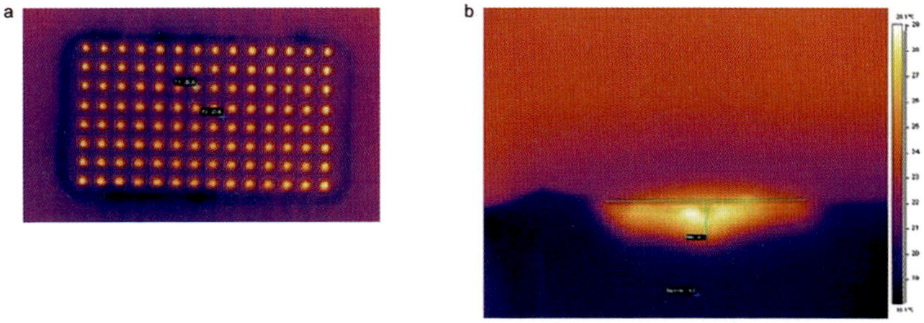

Figure 1 Fractional skin resurfacing. 112 ablation points, 300 micron diameter (a). Simultaneous volumetric heating for anti wrinkles and scar therapy (100% coverage) – Heating (Δ = 18.3° C) to a depth of 2.9 mm – Lab simulation solid organic Gel, recorded live on calibrated FLIR Thermal camera (ThermaCAM SC 640) (setting: 2 W, 70 msec) (b)

tissue is higher than the surrounding tissue, the RF current will be selectively focused to increase heating of the target tissue. Hence, the cooling itself drives electrical current inside the tissue, leading to an increase in penetration depth.

Pixel^{RF} from Alma

It uses a fractionated skin resurfacing module based on UniPolar™ RF-based technology. The Pixel^{RF} tips with Micro Plasma Technology™ create multiple controlled, microperforations within small zones of thermal injury, similar to the pattern created by many fractionated skin resurfacing lasers. The ablative fractional RF module is incorporated into a unipolar RF-based hand-piece. The hand-piece receives RF energy, which includes a stationary tip (12 mm in diameter). An array of protrusions (tiny metal pins) arranged 1 mm apart is configured to cause multiple electrical discharges generated in response to the RF electrical power in a space between the protrusions and the skin. The ablative microplasma RF energy stimulates micro-sparks between the skin surface and RF protrusions, producing holes of 100-150 microns in depth (evaporation + thermal) and 80-120 lm in diameter (width) on the skin surface. During the procedure, just a small portion of the tissue is ablated. The remaining tissue supplies the healing that leads to the elimination of irregular epidermal pigmentation, tightening of dermal collagen and the smoothing that results from the generation of new collagen. The 18 mm width IN-Motion roller tip allows coverage of large areas (full face) in less than 10 minutes. Stationary tips with assorted spot sizes are also available for small, localized areas.

Micro-needles systems

Some devices are based on micro-needles, delivering bipolar RF and now also unipolar RF below the epidermis. One of the first device is the *E prime (Syneron)* for the treatment of skin, creating dermal lesions known as radiofrequency thermal zones. RF thermal zone (RFTZ) patterns in the reticular dermis consist of denatured collagen separated by zones of spared dermis. The FRF system delivers bipolar RF energy to the dermis via 5 micro-needle 30 gauge electrode pairs, 6 mm in length, each spaced 1.25 mm apart. The proximal end of each micro-needle is insulated with a biocompatible Teflon layer, leaving the distal

3 mm exposed to form the electrode in tissue. A thermocouple embedded in the tip of each electrode pair measures tissue temperature during treatment to provide real-time feedback to the generator via a proportional integration derivative (PID) control algorithm.

During RF energy application, the dermal tissue temperature within the RFTZ is maintained at 72° C for 4 seconds using IFS, a proprietary real-time intelligent feedback system allowing to monitor and modulate the fluence and tissue temperature. By varying pulse length, the lesion size is tunable.

One more device belongs to this class, delivering RF with few needles and longer durations sub-epidermally: the intradermal RF device (SpheroFill; PromoItalia Inc., Naples, Italy). This is a bipolar electric wave generator that can emit at two different frequencies (1,134 and 1,769 kHz) within the range of AM broadcasting radio waves (525-1,775 kHz). Bipolar RF is emitted through a needle electrode.

Intracell (Jeisys) uses 49 needles in a stamp with coated needles of 0.5, 0.8, 1.5 or 2 mm in length, emitting either bipolar or unipolar RF below the epidermis after penetrating the skin, called FRM (minimally invasive Fractional Radiofrequency Micro-needles) Fig. 2 and 3. The device gives selective heating in the dermis. Without any epidermal ablation, no wounds or down time occur. However superficial treatment is available by using the 0.5 mm needles.

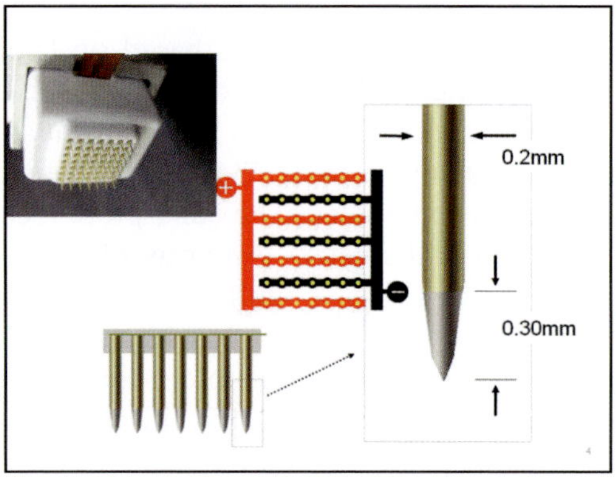

Figure 2 Intracell device

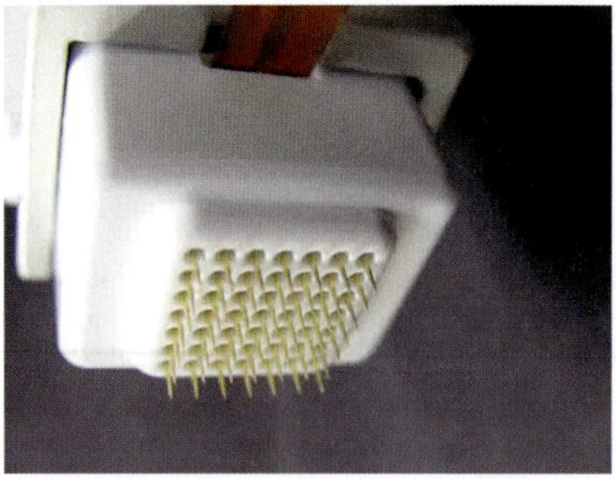

Figure 3 Intracell device, stamp of 49 needles

In addition a newer “SRR” handpiece is available which allows superficial ablation of the epidermis to be performed alone or in combination with deep dermis RF treatment and heating by emission of superficial epidermal bipolar RF. The device gives selective heating in the epidermis without any significant epidermal ablation, no wounds or down time, resulting in improvement without downtime and risk of significant side effects. SRR is an important option for the treatment of facial skin laxity and scars especially in delicate areas such as periorbital, neck lines, frontal area, lips and décolleté.

Deep dermal fractional heating occurs without epidermal wounds. Neo-collagenesis replaces collagen but requires time, the degree of neo-collagenesis depends on the energy levels.

The variety of penetration depths and micro-needles plus the superficial approach with the SRR handpiece allow multilayer treatments according to the indication.

Similar technologies are available from Lutronic or (Scarlet TM, Viol Co., Korea). Scarlet however uses uncoated needles, so the RF is applied to the full length of the needle insertion tunnel and not just at the tip, which might cause more damage to the tissue.

The systems differ in insertion depth of the needles, the fluence that can be applied, uni – or bipolar RF and duration of the RF application.

Compared to a long application of 4 sec with the e-prime, the FRM duration is 0.01 s only. This means that for the long application, intensive – even general – anaesthesia is needed, whereas for FRM topical anaesthesia is sufficient.

A similar RF device is available with *Lutronic* (or *Scarlet TM, Viol Co., Korea*), uses disposable single-use treatment tip consisting of five non-insulated micro-needle electrode pairs per the area of 10 mm^2, with the exposed electrode extending from 0.5 to 3 mm below the skin surface. These bipolar electrode pins form a closed circuit through the irradiated skin, delivering 2 MHz of conducted RF current to the skin. Adjustable RF voltage up to a maximum of 40 V can be delivered, in relation to the intensity (1-10) and conduction time (100-800 ms) (instead of 4 s).

A novel *Micro-needle RF system* (Micro-needle Skin Remodeling Intensif handpiece, *EndyMed Medical*, Caesarea, Israel) for targeted skin rejuvenation for deep, stubborn skin lesions such as acne scars, deep facial wrinkles, striae and dilated pores has been developed. This device uses an array of 25 gold plated tapered micro-needles that penetrate up to 3.5 mm into the skin delivering RF energy to create controlled coagulation zones through the dermis. The tested system proprietary hardware and software allow for the first time constant energy delivery, independent of individual tissue impedance. In contrast to other RF Micro-needle systems on the market, the new Intensif by Endymed handpiece offers enhanced volumetric heating mode with full hemostasis. Clinical studies have shown high efficacy of Endymed’s Micro-needle RF handpiece for skin rejuvenation and especially atrophic acne scars [7] Fig. 4-5.

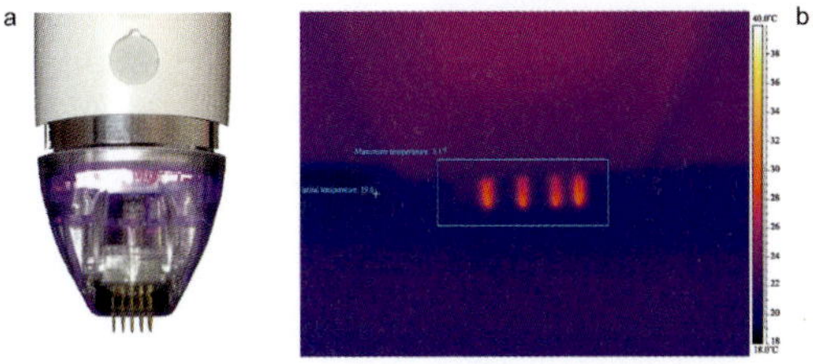

Figure 4 EndyMed’s Intensif Handpiece (a). Thermal image of a treatment of laboratory skin model with impedance similar to dermal impedance (Flir Systems, ThermaCAM SC 640) (b)

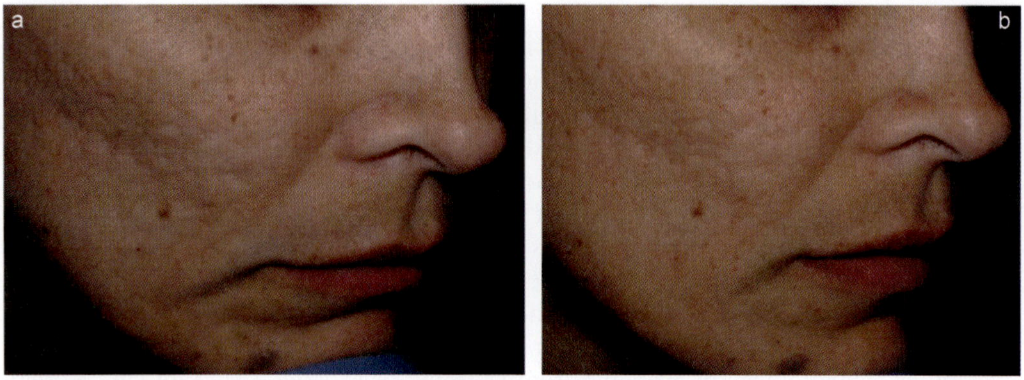

Figure 5 Baseline (a). On month after two micro-needle RF treatments sessions. Decrease in the number and depth of the scars (b)

EFFECTS OF FRACTIONAL RF – WHICH EFFECTS ARE PROVEN?

Superficial bipolar RF Fig. 6

E- Matrix/E-Two Syneron

A bipolar RF-based device delivering RF energy, that is tunable for ablation, coagulation and heating uses the Matrix RF (Syneron) applicator. The thermal effect from RF devices relates to the impedance of skin, not absorption by chromophores as is the case with lasers. As a result, in contrast to columnar or conical zones induced by laser-based fractional systems, the energy that this bipolar RF-based fractional system delivers creates pyramid-shape fractionated thermal zones in the skin. That means, the energy impact is narrower at the epidermal surface and wider and deeper into the dermis [5]. This unique

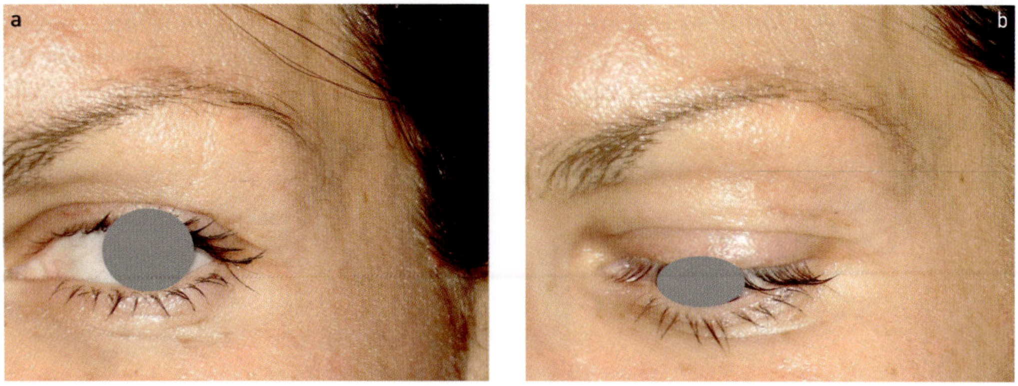

Figure 6 Eye wrinkle before (a) and after one treatment session by fractional RF (b)

lesion geometry provides the main advantage of this modality: volumetric subsurface heating associated with dermal remodeling, with little disruption of epidermis where melanocytes reside [8]. Studies demonstrated that 90% of subjects with skin type II to IV showed improvement in smoothness and wrinkling, 87% in skin tightness, and 83% in skin brightness 1 month after three sublative RF treatments [8].

Six weeks after 3 sessions 4 weeks apart this fractional RF treatment produced moderate (26-50%) and incremental improvements 61%, 35%, 78%, 87%, and 83% subjects achieved more than 50% improvement in fine lines, pores, smoothness and tightness, brightness, and overall appearance, respectively, but did not achieve statistical significance. The degree of elastosis was 5.46 at baseline, which decreased significantly to 4.05 at 6-week follow-up.

The fractional RF treatment was generally well tolerated. Mild erythema developed in most patients for an average of 49.7 hours after irradiation (51.7 hours for first, 53.6 hours for second, 43.9 hours for third session).

73% of patients had 51% to 75% improvement in facial photodamage 9 months after a series of non ablative FP resurfacing [9]. In a comparison study the fractionated bipolar RF device was better tolerated than the fractionated laser with RF [10]. Improvement scores at six weeks did not differ significantly at 55 watts and 75 watts of RF power. At six weeks (for either facial side), approximately 67% of subjects achieved either 25% to 75% or 51% to 75% improvement in fine lines and wrinkles, brightness, tightness, and in overall improvement. Improvement rates were lower for color and pore size. Subjects were either satisfied (67%) or very satisfied (33%) [11].

Superficial (3 DEEP)

Computerized controlled RF (Endymed)

This system generates pulses causing a non-ablative deep dermal heating effect, resulting in simultaneous fractional microablation of the epidermis together with volumetric heating and skin tightening.

Treatment pulses of:

- 62 mJ/pin cause ablation of 200 µm and coagulation depth up to 300 µm;
- 40 mJ/pin cause ablation of 150 µm and coagulation depth up to 200 µm;
- 20 mJ/pin cause ablation of 80 µm and coagulation depth up to 120 µm.

Small coagulative thermal lesions are surrounded by undamaged epidermal tissue.

Three treatments, 4 weeks apart, result in significant reduction in the depth of wrinkles and acne scars after 3 months [12].

Specimen slides taken immediately after treatment revealed the degree of improvement is moderate to good (25-75% improvement) in most treated patients. These results support significant improvement in skin texture as a result of the treatment 4 weeks after therapy with further improvement after 3 months [13]. After six sessions (the first 4 sessions at 2-week intervals and 2 sessions at 3-week intervals), a greater degree of clinical improvement was found in patients with surface temperature greater than 11.5 C increase at the end of the procedure and remaining greater than 4.5 C 20 minutes later Fig. 7. Changes induced by radiofrequency show structural improvements at the dermal-epidermal junction using confocal microscopy [14].

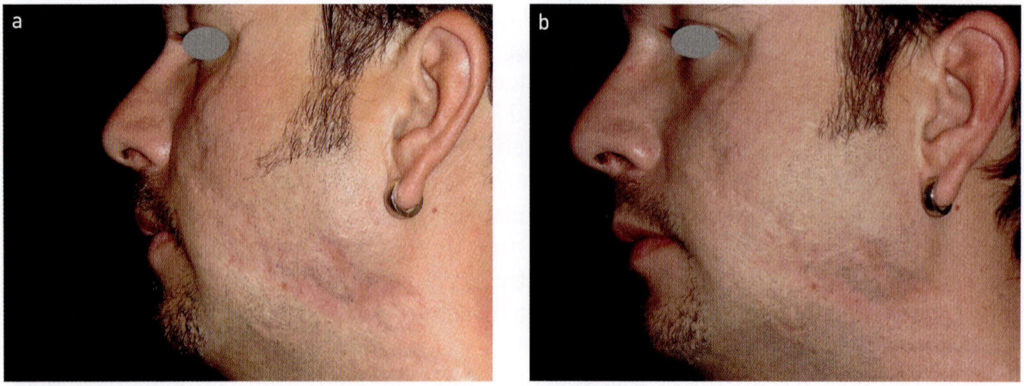

Figure 7 Cutaneous scars before (a) and after 6 sessions of treatment by Endymed (1 month between each session) (b)

Plasma

The handpiece of a microplasma radiofrequency device, using an array of closely applied microperforations in the skin, produces a series of closely spaced spicules, which contact the skin and provide a thin air gap between the skin surface and the roof of the electrode. The discharge of radiofrequency energy at a small distance from the skin forms plasma, a state of matter in which a portion of the molecules is ionized. Because plasma is sensitive to electromagnetic fields, the radiofrequency current triggers microsparks in the plasma between the skin surface and the electrode spicules. These sparks cause mild epidermal ablation and perforate the dermis superficially to form microchannels [15].

Micro-needle delivered RF

Endymed

One of the first RF technologies scientifically evaluated is the bipolar FRF system that delivers bipolar RF energy to the dermis via 5 micro-needles (Syneron E Prime) creating RF thermal zones (RFTZ). Patterns in the reticular dermis consist of denatured collagen separated by zones of spared dermis.

Hantash *et al.* studied the effect of RF due to duration: results simulating a 70° C target temperature treatment with a pulse duration of 5 seconds. Tissue temperature after 1 second of RF application was measured at 67° C, and 2 seconds later reached the target temperature of 70° C without overshoot. Tissue had cooled to 55° C 1 second following energy delivery.

In a dermal thickness of 2 mm 95.7% of the power was deposited in the dermal layer, 2.3% in the subcutaneous, and 2.0% in the epidermal layer [16].

RF thermal zone (RFTZ) pattern in the reticular dermis consisted of zones of denatured collagen separated by zones of spared dermis through day 28 post-treatment, then replaced by new dermal tissue by 10 weeks.

HSP72 expression rapidly diminished after day 2, while HSP47 expression increased progressively through 10 weeks.

Reticular dermal volume, cellularity, hyaluronic acid, and elastin content increased. RT-PCR studies revealed an immediate increase in IL-1b, TNF-a, and MMP-13, whereas MMP-1, HSP72, HSP47, and TGF-b levels increased by 2 days. A marked induction of tropoelastin, fibrillin, as well as procollagens 1 and 3 was observed by 28 days post-treatment. This demonstrates a significant wound healing response and an active dermal remodeling process with new collagen by 10 weeks post-treatment, and proves a profound neoelastogenesis following RF treatment of human skin [17].

A clinical study compared facial skin laxity treatment with this RF technology to results following surgical face-lift.

Blinded grading of photographs demonstrated a statistically significant 49% improvement in skin laxity relative to baseline for the surgical facelift, compared with 16% for FRF. The surgical face-lift resulted in a mean 1.20-grade improvement on the 4-point laxity grading scale. The mean laxity improvement from a single FRF treatment was 37% that of the surgical face-lift. Patient satisfaction was high, participants in the FRF treatment group experienced only mild transient erythema or edema [18].

Changes in objective measurements of mechanical skin properties were studied by one group. Three months after treatment, elastometry measurements showed statistically significant improvement (5-12% decrease in Young's Modulus and 10-16% decrease in retraction time) and at 3 months showed a statistically significant improvement of 1.42 grades on the Fitzpatrick scale for wrinkles, and 0.66 grades on the Alexiades scale for skin laxity, increasing to 1.57 and 0.70 improvement, respectively, at 6 months. Eighty-nine percent and 91% of patients were satisfied or very satisfied with the procedure [19].

Endymed's Intensif micro-needle fractional RF handpiece was used in a recent clinical study. This handpiece uses a tip with 25 non-insulated, gold plated micro-needle electrodes. The needles are inserted into the skin by a specially designed electronically controlled, smooth motion motor minimizing patient discomfort. RF emission delivered over the whole dermal portion of the needle allows effective coagulation resulting in minimal or no bleeding, together with bulk volumetric heating. The study included 20 patients, treated for depressed acne scars. The degree of clinical improvement was assessed by the global aesthetic improvement scale (GAIS) and subjects satisfaction by post treatment questionnaires.

Results: the number of treatments per patient varied between 1 and 6 (average 3.3 treatments per patient). Eleven patients (55%) reported none to minimal pain, 6 (30%) moderate discomfort and only 3 (15%) reported significant pain. Objective evaluation of the improvement by a board certified dermatologist showed improvement in 95% of patients. 25% showed excellent improvement, 50% experienced good improvement, and the 20% showed minimal improvement. One patient showed no improvement [20].

Anaesthesia

According to practitioners using this system, the treatment needs complete local anaesthesia or even more, whereas other systems with shorter duration of RF delivery can be done under topical anaesthesia.

Mostly topical 4% lidocaine cream is applied about 30 minutes before the procedure. An epidermal cooling device (CARESYS, Danil SMC, Korea) was used to relieve pain and erythema after the treatment.

Intracell Fig. 8 and 9

This device delivers bipolar radiofrequency energy through 49 micro-needle electrodes in an area of 1 cm^2 into the deep dermis with needle electrodes that are nonconductive, except the tip, which delivers RF. Compared to the E Prime the duration of RF is very short – instead of a fixed 4 sec, the radiofrequency energy delivery durations differ according to energy levels [20].

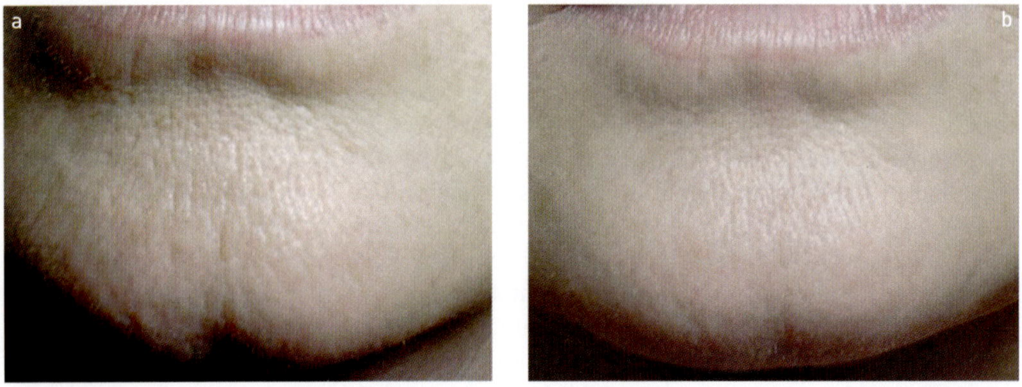

Figure 8 Chin, before (a) and after 3 sessions of Intracell treatment (b)

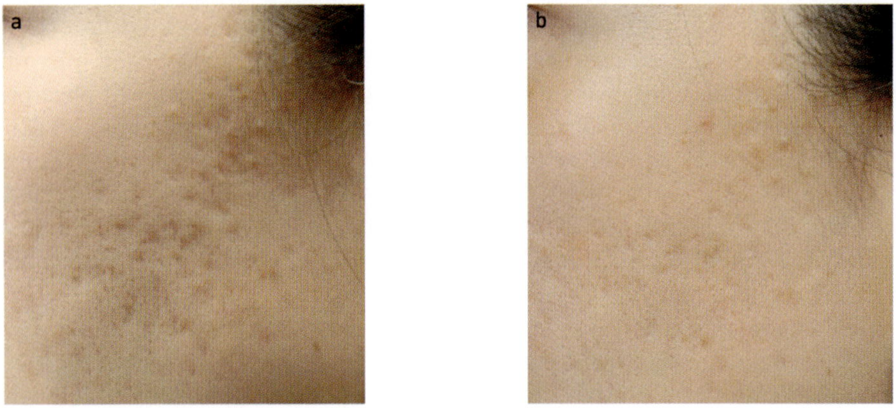

Figure 9 Acne scars before (a) and after 4 sessions of Intracell treatment (1 month between each session) (b)

The grade of acne scars and Investigator Global Assessment of large pores improve in more than 70% of cases. Skin surface roughness, dermal density, and microscopic and composite images also improved, whereas TEWL and sebum measurement do not change. Eight weeks after two sessions of FRM treatment, the grade of acne scars improves in 73.3% of patients, but does not change in 23.3%. Pain persisted for longer than 1 day in 10 patients (33.3%) and for longer than 3 days in five (16.7%). Enlarged pores improve in 70%, do not change in seven cases (23.3%), and aggravated in 6.7%.

Folliculitis was observed in two patients (6.7%), but these lesions were mostly mild. Patient satisfaction at 12 weeks of follow-up was very high in 12 patients (40%), high in 14 (46.7%), ordinary in three (10%). Dermal density decreased 2 and 6 weeks after the 2-week treatment and increased 4 and 8 weeks after the 4-week treatment.

Exclusion criteria should be:

– systemic diseases (e.g., hematologic diseases with bleeding tendency or diabetes mellitus and atopic dermatitis affecting wound healing);
– anticoagulants or antiplatelet agents;
– pregnancy or lactation;
– previous history of frequent herpes simplex viral infection;
– any aesthetic procedures on the face within 6 months prior to the study;
– any implantable electronic device (e.g., pacemaker);
– active infection;
– previous history of hypersensitivity to anaesthetic creams;
– photosensitivity;
– a history of hypertrophic or keloidal scarring;
– the use of isotretinoin within 6 months.

Periorbital wrinkles treated with FRM 3 times at 4 week intervals, using needles – 0.8 mm depth – 12.5 W/100 msec (Intracell TM, Jeysis, Korea), stamping up to 10 times the periorbital area showed 50% improvement, 35% much improvement, 14% very much improvement without significant adverse reaction.

Among the main advantages over fractional lasers is the low risk of PIH.

The powerful thermal damage of deep dermis with perfect epidermal preservation compared to other ablative or non-ablative or fractional laser devices, the very short down time and rare post-treatment complication.

A novel RF system (Micro-needle Skin Remodeling (MFSR) from EndyMed Medical, Israel) for targeted skin rejuvenation also showed significant improvement after 2 sessions and after 4 and 12 weeks follow up in a preliminary study in 2013. All experienced mild to moderate edema, and erythema was documented. Edema resolved after up to 24 hours post treatment and erythema lasted up to 3 days. Invisible micro-ablation in the form of skin roughness was reported up to 3 days post treatment [21].

A similar system, that uses uncoated needles (Scarlet, Korea), was used in 3 consecutive sessions at 4-week intervals using needle penetration depth parameters according to underlying tissue thickness (periorbital area: 0.5 mm, forehead: 0.8 mm, chin and temple: 1 mm, and cheek: 2 mm) giving single, non-overlapping passes.

56% of patients had achieved more than 50% improvement in overall appearance. The mean melanin index (MI) and erythema index (EI) obtained by Mexameter decreased from 77.66 and 296.38 at baseline to 72.26 and 265.66 after the final session. The mean R2 (maximum roughness) and R3 (average roughness) values measured by Visiometer decreased from 0.63 and 1.00 at baseline to 0.55 and 0.85 after the final session (respectively, $P < 0.05$). A significant increase in dermal collagen content was observed at 4 weeks after three sessions of fractional RF compared to the baseline. Immuno-histochemical staining for fibrillin-1 revealed a significant increase in its density from DEJ to the deep dermis compared to the baseline [3].

COMBINATIONS WITH FRACTIONAL RF

Use of fractional laser followed by fractional RF was shown to be safe and effective for acne scars with modest improvement and low PIH rate comparable to other resurfacing techniques in this Asian case series [10].

Drug delivery

Transepidermal drug delivery using ablative fractional technology disrupts the stratum corneum, overcoming the barrier presented for drug penetration. Fractional RF ablation can also be used in that way.

Treatment with fractional RF plus stem cell conditioned medium in 3 sessions at 4-week intervals showed clinical improvement on physician's global assessment and patient satisfaction scores on both the RF only side as well as on the combination with stem cells. Stem cell conditioned medium provided a synergistic effect on improvement of skin roughness, which was statistically significant ($p < 0.05$). Histologic examination revealed marked increase in dermal thickness and dermal collagen content [22].

Three sessions of intradermal RF at intervals of four weeks (1,134 kHz frequency, 12 W power, 26 G electrode size) combined with autologous PRP for striae distensae showed 5.3% excellent, 36.8% marked, 31.6% moderate improvement in Asians [23].

Hypertrophic scars were treated with triamcinolone using fractional ablative RF (Alma fractional RF) combined with an acoustic pressure ultrasound module for acoustic pressure with vibrational cycles ("push-pull") on the skin surface to enhance delivery of the triamcinolone.

The treatment procedure comprised three steps:

- ablative fractional RF for skin perforation;
- topical application of triamcinolone acetonide 20 mg/ml on the perforated skin;
- acoustic pressure wave applied to enhance triamcinolone penetration into the skin.

Complete resolution was seen after one session in patients with scars on the nose and mandibular area. The scar on the neck showed complete resolution after four sessions. The scar on the knee showed a marked improvement after four sessions. Mild and homogeneous atrophy was observed in hypertrophic scars on the neck [24].

Clinical assessment demonstrated significant improvement in the appearance of Striae distensae treated in the same way but using retinoic acid 0.05% compared to little improvement when treated without the cream [25].

CONCLUSION

In summary fractional RF can achieve significant results but those differ widely according to intensity, fluence, heat and duration. Side effets, especially pigmentary changes, are usually less than in chromophore related lasers. The technology is still quite young and numerous new devices, combinations and modifications will be reported in the near future.

REFERENCES

[1] Atiyeh BS, Dibo SA. Nonsurgical nonablative treatment of aging skin: radiofrequency technologies between aggressive marketing and evidence-based efficacy. Aesth Plast Surg 2009; 33: 283-294.

[2] Sadick NS, Makino Y. Selective Electro-thermolysis in Aesthetic Medicine: A Review. Lasers Surg Med 2004; 34: 91-97.

[3] Alster TS, Lupton JR. Nonablative cutaneous remodeling using radiofrequency devices. Clin Dermatol 2007; 25: 487-491.

[4] Elman M, Vider I, Harth Y, Gottfried V, Shemer A. Non invasive therapy of wrinkles, lax skin using a novel multisource phase controlled radiofrequency system. J Cosm Laser Ther 2010; 12: 81-86.

[5] Brightman L, Goldman MP, Taub AF. Sublative rejuvenation: experience with a new fractional radio-frequency system for skin rejuvenation and repair. J Drugs Dermatol 2009; 8: 9-13.

[6] Elman M, Harth Y. Novel Multi-Source Phase-Controlled Radiofrequency Technology for Nonablative and Micro-Ablative Treatment of Wrinkles, Lax Skin and Acne Scars. Laser Therapy 2011; Vol. 20, N° 2, p. 139-144.

[7] Harth Y, Elman M, Ackerman E, Frank I. Depressed acne scars – effective, minimal downtime treatment with a novel smooth motion non-insulated micro-needle radiofrequency technology. J Cosm Dermatol Sci App 2014; 4: 212-218.

[8] Lee HS, Lee DH, *et al.* Fractional rejuvenation using a novel bipolar radiofrequency system in asian skin. Dermatol Surg 2011; 37: 1611-1619.

[9] Willey A, Kilmer S, Newman J, Renton B, *et al.* Elastometry and clinical results after bipolar radiofrequency treatment of skin. Dermatol Surg 2010; 36: 877-884.

[10] Peterson JD, Palm MD, Kiripolsky MG, Guiha I, Goldman MP. Evaluation of the effect of fractional laser with radiofrequency and fractionated radiofrequency on the improvement of acne scars. Dermatol Surg 2011; 37: 1260-1267.

[11] Gold MH, Foster A, Biron JA. Treatment of photoaged skin by fractional bipolar radiofrequency energy Poster EADV 2010.

[12] Sadick Ns, Sato M, Palmisano D, Frank I, Cohen H, Harth Y. In vivo animal histology and clinical evaluation of multisource fractional radiofrequency skin resurfacing (FSR) applicator. J Cosm Laser Ther 2011; 13: 204-209.

[13] Harth Y MD, Fritz K. Treatment of depressed acne scars and deep wrinkles with a novel multisource fractional radiofrequency device – histological and clinical results on 50 patients with long term follow-up Poster, Aslms 2011.

[14] Royo Torre De La Jr, Moreno-Moraga J, Estefania Muñoz E, Cornejo Navarro P. Multisource, Phase-controlled radiofrequency for treatment of skin laxity correlation between clinical and in-vivo confocal microscopy results and real-time thermal changes. J Clin Aesthet Dermatol 2011; 4(1): 28-35.

[15] Halachmi S, Orenstein A, Meneghel T, *et al.* A novel fractional micro-plasma radio-frequency technology for the treatment of facial scars and rhytids: a pilot study. J Cosmet Laser Therapy 2010; 12: 208-212.

[16] Hantash BM, Renton B, Berkowitz RL, Stridde BC, *et al.* Pilot clinical study of a novel minimally invasive bipolar micro-needle radiofrequency device. Lasers Surg Med 2009b; 41: 87-95.

[17] Hantash BM, Ubeid AA, Chang H, Kafi R, *et al.* Bipolar fractional radiofrequency treatment induces neoelastogenesis and neocollagenesis. Lasers Surg Med 2009a; 41: 1-9.

[18] Alexiades-Armenakas M, Rosenberg D, Renton B, Dover J, Arndt K. Blinded, randomized, quantitative grading comparison of minimally invasive, fractional radiofrequency and surgical face-lift to treat skin laxity. Arch Dermatol 2010; 146(4): 396-405.

[19] Cho Si, Chung BY, Choi Mg, Baek JH, *et al.* Evaluation of the clinical efficacy of fractional radio-frequency micro-needle treatment in acne scars and large facial pores. Dermatol Surg 2012; 38: 1017-1024.

[20] Harth Y, *et al.* Depressed acne scars-effective, minimal downtime treatment with a novel smooth motion non-insulated micro-needle radiofrequency technology. J Cosm Dermatol Sci Appl 2014; 4: 212-218.

[21] Fritz K. Presentation 5. Congress Cannes 2013.

[22] Seo KY, Yoon MS, Kim DH, Lee HJ. Skin rejuvenation by micro-needle fractional radiofrequency treatment in asian skin; clinical and histological analysis. Lasers Surg Med 2012; 44: 631-636.

[23] Kim IS, Park KY, Kim BJ, Kim MN, Kim CW, Kim SE. Efficacy of intradermal radiofrequency combined withautologous platelet-rich plasma in striae distensae: a pilot study. Int J Dermatol 2012; 51: 1253-1258.

[24] Issa MCA, Kassuga LEBP, Chevrand NS, Pires MT. Topical delivery of triamcinolone via skin pretreated with ablative radiofrequency: a new method in hypertrophic scar treatment. Int J Dermatol 2013; 52: 367-370.

[25] Issa MCA, de Britto LE, Kassuga, P, Stroligo N, *et al.* Transepidermal retinoic acid delivery using ablative fractional radiofrequency associated with acoustic pressure ultrasound for stretch marks treatment. Lasers Surg Med 2013; 45: 81-88.

CHAPTER 9

Microfocused ultrasound

Jean-Michel Mazer

Microfocused ultrasound is a new technique for managing facial rejuvenation that is indicated to treat the laxity of the facial outline and possibly of the lower eyelid. It presents specific characteristics that are unique to ultrasound beams. It differs from other laser and radiofrequency techniques in its ability to act on very deep tissue, reaching as far as the deepest structures of the skin, the subcutaneous tissue and the superficial muscular aponeurotic system.

CHARACTERISTICS OF MICROFOCUSED ULTRASOUND

The medical usage of ultrasound has been widely known for many years, especially in the context of medical imaging where it is known as sonography. If very high powers are used, ultrasound can have a thermal effect. The characteristics of ultrasound in terms of the action on tissue depend on the frequency of the emission, the power of the system, and whether or not the beams are focused. One well-known imaging technique that uses high-frequency ultrasound beams of around 20 MHz on the skin is called high-resolution sonography for skin imaging. There are medical applications currently using ultrasound beams that are based on the induction of a powerful and deep thermal effect. These systems can be used to treat liver and breast tumours, which are located using sonography and then targeted with very high-power doses, producing a thermal effect that is intended to destroy the tumour. This is made possible by the principle of focused ultrasound.

Principle of focused ultrasound

The principle of focused ultrasound can be compared to setting fire to a sheet of paper using only a magnifying glass and the energy from the sun's rays. Ultrasound beams are emitted over a relatively large surface area but they are fully focused on a specific point, known as the focal point, which is relatively deep. They converge and concentrate on the focal point. On the surface and beyond this focal point, due to the lack of ultrasound convergence, the effect is very weak. However, at the point where the ultrasound beams converge, because of the phenomenon of concentration, the power is very high and this leads to a significant rise in temperature.

In dermatology, ultrasound beams are already used to produce lipolysis in the subcutaneous tissue (panniculus adiposus). This can be done with high-intensity focused ultrasound: Liposonix™ (Solta). This treatment consists of a powerful thermal effect leading to some degree of adipocyte lysis, which is followed by neocollagen synthesis that fights laxity.

By contrast, the use of lower frequency ultrasound can trigger vibratory phenomena affecting adipocyte membranes. These membranes are more fragile than those of other cells, so this process triggers adipocyte rupture, an effect that is mechanical rather than thermal. This technique is used in focused ultrasound systems such as Ultrashape™.

If the aim is to exert a thermal effect on the deepest layers of the dermis, the subcutaneous tissue, and indeed the SMAS (superficial muscular aponeurotic system), the thermal effect will be powerful enough to lead to tissue coagulation, which in turn causes neocollagen synthesis and retraction of structures that are high in collagen. This is what is used in microfocused systems (Ulthera™). With this technique, studies have demonstrated that tissue coagulation lesions are created following an extremely significant temperature elevation to 64° C [1, 2]. This triggers the retraction and then the synthesis of collagen fibres. Depending on the choice of transducer and the frequency used (the higher the ultrasound frequency, the less significant the depth of penetration achieved), it is therefore possible to target structures located 1.5 mm, 3 mm (subcutaneous tissue), or even 4.5 mm deep, as far as the SMAS.

This is the only technology that has been approved to this date for facial and neck rejuvenation.

Main indications for microfocused ultrasound

The two main indications for microfocused ultrasound in facial rejuvenation are treatment of the eyelids and the facial outline:

– for the facial outline, the targeted areas are under the chin, the top of the neck, the jowls and outer cheeks, and possibly the area behind the nasolabial folds. It is crucial to avoid the ultrasound beams reaching bone structures. This is possible with anatomic knowledge and it can be confirmed, if doubts persist, by real-time use of sonography that is incorporated into this system;

– when treating the face, only the mandibular border needs to be avoided; for the neck, care must be exercised to avoid the cartilage of the larynx; for the forehead, the usual depth targeted varies from three to five millimetres. This means that sonographical skin imaging can be carried out using the system. If the depth does not exceed three millimetres, only a single depth of action should be used (3 mm), and the 4.5 mm depth transducer cannot be used.

The treatment consists of aligning the points of impact side by side in order to treat the whole area [3]. Some other areas must be avoided, especially the chin area and underneath the labial commissures, to avoid inducing a tightening of the labial commissures, which would trigger the beginnings of marionette lines. The treated areas will mainly be those under the chin and the jaw, as well as the jowls. This leads to an improved facial outline.

If there is a desire for correction of loose eyebrows, the forehead will be treated, especially the lateral area, as the aim should be to treat the outer end of the eyebrow rather than the inner section. To achieve a lifting effect on a loose eyebrow, the superior part, the area below the eyebrow, and the eyelids are treated.

In all cases, it is crucial to ensure that the treatment never reaches the bone structures (frontal bone, malar bone, mandible) and cartilaginous structures (larynx). If there is any doubt, the sonographic imaging function that is incorporated into the Ulthera system will allow the practitioner to see the exact depths of the cutaneous structures and the proximity of bones or cartilage. Wherever possible, the aim is to perform two successive passes, the first being 4.5 mm deep and the second at 3 mm, which should always be achievable when treating the facial outline.

The theoretical risk of reaching a facial nerve branch can readily be overcome since in the areas suitable for this treatment, the most superficial branches of the facial nerve are located at depths of greater than 9 mm, and the deepest point targeted with this treatment will not exceed 4.5 mm.

A USEFUL QUALITY OF ULTRASOUND REGARDING THE CUTANEOUS PHOTOTYPE

In contrast to laser treatments, ultrasound beams are not sensitive to melanin. There is no absorption, or interaction with epidermal melanin. The inflammatory reaction occurs at a level too deep to entail any risk of post-inflammatory hyperpigmentation. This means that the treatment is the same for all phototypes and irrespective of current tan.

RECOVERY FROM TREATMENT

Due to the significant depth of action, with no reaction at the surface because of ultrasound focusing, recovery is extremely straightforward, usually consisting only of transient erythema that does not last beyond 15 minutes.

In rare cases [4-7] there is oedema of the eyelids or, if the upper eyelid is treated, reduced sensation in the forehead that persists for several days but is always reversible. Some superficial ecchymoses covering a small surface area may also be seen, and there may be increased pain in the area under the chin or in the eyelids that persists for a few days. There is no need for patients to avoid social contact. No significant or problematic side effect has been reported in any of the various studies. A recent personal study [8] taking in 233 cases highlighted the safety of this method.

In practical terms, no additional care is needed after the session.

DISADVANTAGES

The main disadvantage of this method is that it is relatively painful, which means that the patient needs to be quite motivated to proceed. This is because the deep focal points, which undergo a temperature elevation to 64° C, can trigger fleeting burning sensations. Furthermore, there is no suitable anaesthesia to offer because anaesthetic creams do not act deeply enough to be effective, and lidocaine injections are too high in water to be considered since there would be an interaction between the water injected with the xylocaine and the ultrasound beams. This means that the only anaesthesia that can be offered is a prescription of oral ibuprofen and paracetamol one hour before the session. Further anaesthesia is achieved using "small actions", specifically oral pain-relief and the use of vibrating devices to distract the brain.

For patients who ultimately cannot tolerate the pain, which in practice occurs very rarely, it is possible to offer ambulatory inhalation anaesthesia with nitrous oxide.

INDICATIONS AND EFFICACY

Due to the extremely deep action of microfocused ultrasound, compared to lasers and radiofrequency, there is a major tightening effect. This means that it is indicated for the treatment of laxity in the two areas that are particularly prone to benefit from it Fig. 1. This is even more noteworthy considering that genuine alternatives to surgery in these areas, the outline of the face and the upper eyelids, were previously unavailable. Therefore the two main indications are the treatment of the facial outline and upper eyelid laxity. The results can usually be seen after one session. Evidence shows that while microfocused ultrasound is not as effective as a true surgical lifting procedure, results are generally very clear from the first session. In general the patient is offered a single session. If there is very severe looseness or more noticeable fatty deposits, a second session can be offered in order to heighten the results. For the upper eyelid, a second session is more common, given that there is only a small skin surface area that can be targeted by ultrasound beams; a second treatment must be considered in around half of all cases.

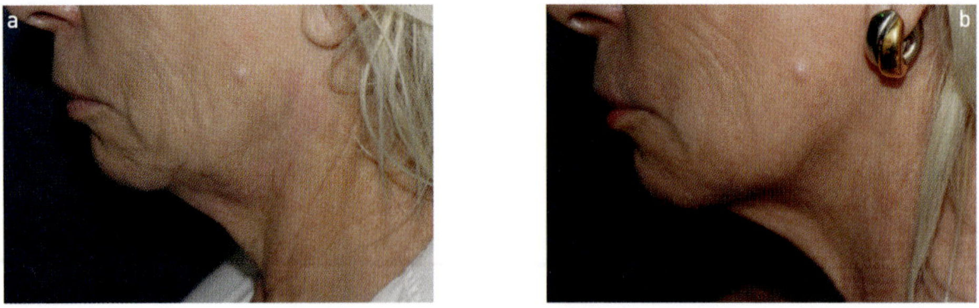

Figure 1 Example of results on the facial outline
(a) Before and 3 months after a session of microfocused ultrasound: the result in the submandibular area and the superior lateral neck is clearer than in the jowls, which are always more difficult to improve (b)

CONCLUSION

Microfocused ultrasound is a new technique that is especially useful for managing facial rejuvenation since it addresses a problem that has until now been difficult to treat except with a surgical lift: loosening of the facial outline. While it may not be as effective as a surgical lift, the results are still clearly visible. Recovery is relatively straightforward, and the main drawback is that the treatment is quite painful; the patient will accept this, however, if they are sufficiently motivated.

REFERENCES

[1] Laubach HJ, *et al.* Intense focused ultrasound: evaluation of a new treatment modality for precise microcoagulation within the skin. Dermatol Surg 2008; 34(5): 727-734.

[2] Gliklich RE, *et al.* Clinical pilot study of intense ultrasound therapy to deep dermal facial skin and subcutaneous tissues. Arch Facial Plast Surg 2007; 9(2): 88-95.

[3] Chan NP, *et al.* Safety study of transcutaneous focused ultrasound for non-invasive skin tightening in Asians. Lasers Surg Med 2011; 43(5): 366-375.

[4] Weiss M. Commentary: noninvasive skin tightening: ultrasound and other technologies: where are we? Dermatol Surg 2012; 38(1): 28-30.

[5] Alam M, *et al.* Ultrasound tightening of facial and neck skin: a rater-blinded prospective cohort study. J Am Acad Dermatol 2010; 62(2): 262-269.

[6] Lee HS, *et al.* Multiple pass ultrasound tightening of skin laxity of the lower face and neck. Dermatol Surg 2011.

[7] Suh DH, *et al.* Intense focused ultrasound tightening in asian skin: clinical and pathologic results. Dermatol Surg 2011; 37(11): 1595-1602.

[8] Mazer JM, *et al.* Tolérance des ultrasons microfocalisés. A propos de 230 traitements. Congrès des JDIP, Paris, 16 juin 2013.

CHAPTER 10

Facial rejuvenation: other techniques

Jean-Luc Vigneron

CHEMICAL PEELS

Introduction

The quest for beautiful skin and a clear, radiant complexion has been ongoing for countless years and has for the most part predated photon-based technologies. In this chapter we will discuss previous rejuvenation techniques and more recent techniques that do not use light or radiofrequency energy.

Chemical peels

Peels make use of the effects of chemical substances on the cutaneous tissue with the aim of stimulating synthesis of elastin and collagen fibres. Their clinical effects are so obvious that there are very few studies on the quantitative and qualitative effects of chemical peels on dermatoheliosis. The so-called "reversal" effect is widely known, and the long-standing existence of chemical peels (Egypt, 3,000 years BC) has given them a permanent place in the arsenal of rejuvenation techniques.

The rare studies on chemical peels are demonstrative. Histological studies of a number of cases carried out by Stegman [1] in the 1980s compared, on the same person, skin that had undergone a deep phenol peel more than 20 years ago with neighbouring untreated skin. The treated skin showed a denser dermis, with longer fibre structures present in greater numbers, presenting a better and more horizontal arrangement. They showed that the epidermis presents improved thickness, equating an increased surface area for dermoepidermal exchange, and thus improved mitotic activity in the *stratum basale*.

Butler's histochemical studies [2] showed that medium and deep peels induce a renewed and thickened dermis containing collagen and glycosaminoglycans in identical percentages to that of the control tissue from a young subject. This is genuine rejuvenation!

Chemical peeling agents were applied to the back of 100 irradiated mice. Histology was carried out using standard and polarised light microscopes in order to measure the thickness of the dermis, and the appearance and organisation of collagen and elastin. Specimens were used to quantify glycosaminoglycan and collagen content per unit volume [2].

P. Butler's study demonstrated that *all peels* produced reorganisation of dermal collagen and an increase in birefringence, especially in the papillary dermis. They also eradicated the elastotic masses in the dermis considered to be pathognomonic of dermatoheliosis, and reorganised elastic fibres into a network of fine horizontal fibrils with far fewer vertical fibrils.

In the 33% TCA peels and especially the phenol peels, this new organised network of elastic fibres was also present in the deeper layers of the reticular dermis.

The results of this study suggest that the clinical effects of chemical peels are caused by at least two mechanisms in the dermis: structural reorganisation and increased volume. Fibroblast function seems to be the target of chemical peels.

Indications for chemical peels (see table)

	Superficial peel Fig. 1	Medium peel Fig. 2	Deep peel Fig. 3	Specific hormonal spot peel Fig. 4
Recommended products	AHA: glycolic acid, mandelic acid, lactic acid, pyruvic acid BHA: salicylic acid, TCA-C (trichloroacetic acid cream system) max 15-18%	TCA (trichloroacetic acid) 20-30%. Max 30% weight by weight TCA lotion, clay-based formula, very safe	Phenol Croton oil	Idebenone Mandelic acid Emblica Retinoic acid
To be avoided	pH too low Intervention performed too slowly	Low% of phenol, no more effective than TCA, but with prolonged redness	Trichloroacetic acid due to a risk of scarring Non-homogenous phenol formulations	Trichloroacetic acid due to hyperpigmentation
Disadvantages	If glycolic acid is used, very close monitoring is required	Inherent risk in medium peels: hyperpigmentation	Prolonged redness for several months with phototypes 0 and 1	?
Side effects	Epidermolysisif a low pH product is used or application is to weakened skin Rare cases of sebaceous growths	Irregular result if not applied evenly	Transient telangiectasiaand folliculitis, hypopigmentation in phototypes 1 and 2 if very wrinkled Hypertrophic scars on skin that has few pilosebaceous units Beware of "hand made" formulations	Results are sometimes insufficient on longstanding melasma. In this case, a phenol peel is advised

	Superficial peel Fig. 1	Medium peel Fig. 2	Deep peel Fig. 3	Specific hormonal spot peel Fig. 4
Patient experience	A few minutes of tingling	Intense heat during the peel (20 minutes)	100% lack of sensation during the peel. Intense heating 60% of cases from the 3rd to the 6th hour. 1 week of discomfort but no more	A few minutes of tingling
Recovery	AHA and BHA: redness for a few minutes, no desquamation TCA-C: very fine desquamation No social discomfort	6 days: initial brown discolouration followed by frank desquamation Effective for three years	24 hours of occlusive dressing 7 days of face powder 4-6 weeks of sensitivity 10 years of satisfaction	Fine desquamation
Sequence	3 peels at 2-3 week intervals	One peel, sometimes with an additional "retouch" the following day	One peel lasting 1 hr 30 Obligatory targeted retouch the following day to ensure an even result	Peel Application of a specific cream every day for 21 days Then on D21, check-up and 2nd peelif necessary
Indications	AHA: Brighten complexion Dermatoheliosis 1 BHA: Seborrhoea and acne TCA-C: Dermatoheliosis 1 and 2	Dermatoheliosis 2 and 3	All wrinkles Dermatoheliosis 3 with a thickened stratum corneum Dermatoheliosis 4 Cheek ptosis All pigmented lesions Eyelid laxity Acne and post-traumatic scars	Melasma, even longstanding, even resistant
Durability	3 peels at 2-week intervals will have an effect lasting 6 months	2-4 years depending on sun exposure, tobacco use, and use of cosmetic stimulants	7-15 years, withperiorbital and perioral wrinkles returning, but always less severely than before the peel. Treated cheeks seem to resist further change	No recurrence of melasma if it remains suppressed for a full year
Contraindications	Allergy to glycolic acid (very unusual)	Active herpes	Active herpes Poorly controlled diabetes	Active herpes Melasma in which the hormonal cause is still present

	Superficial peel Fig. 1	Medium peel Fig. 2	Deep peel Fig. 3	Specific hormonal spot peel Fig. 4
Ease of execution for the doctor	Act quickly Monitor The stopwatch is not the greatest ally	Act quickly Monitor Check that the area of frosting required is even	A phenol peel is acompetitive techniquethat can have a lot to offer. Training is necessary Standard learning curve at first, but the improvement in quality of the results seems to be limitless Local anaesthetic only with monitoring	Very easy
Particularities	AHA: The clay-based form of glycolic acid can be used to treat unprepared skin: starter peel. BHA: salicylic acid is able to treat acne due to sebum retention TCA-C: TCA15 or 18 followed by the specific cream are visibly more effective than glycolic treatments	Prepare the skin in order to avoid hyperpigmentation	Baker-Gordon: always causes achromia Hetter peel: clever but difficult to prepare Exopeel: only homogenous and clear formula that does not need to be stirred Progressive formula	60% very good immediate results Needs specific maintenance treatmentafter several months to be gradually spaced out Rejuvenating effect on the whole face
Possible combinations of techniques	Alternating LED Toxins and fillers can be used the same day	Toxin before treatment for a less mobile face during re-epithelialisation Lip line fillers Fillers performed during the peel last longer	Toxin a few days before for a less mobile face during re-epithelialisation Lip line fillers Fillers performed during the peel last longer Before and during, manual or microRF needling for scars	Toxin and fillers can be used the same day
Combinations of deep peels with different actions: combined peel		Deep phenol peel on very wrinkled areas Medium TCA 30 peel on the rest of the face If two peels with different actions are used, there must be differing levels of dermatoheliosis On a face with uniform dermatoheliosis 4, a combined peel will never be offered		

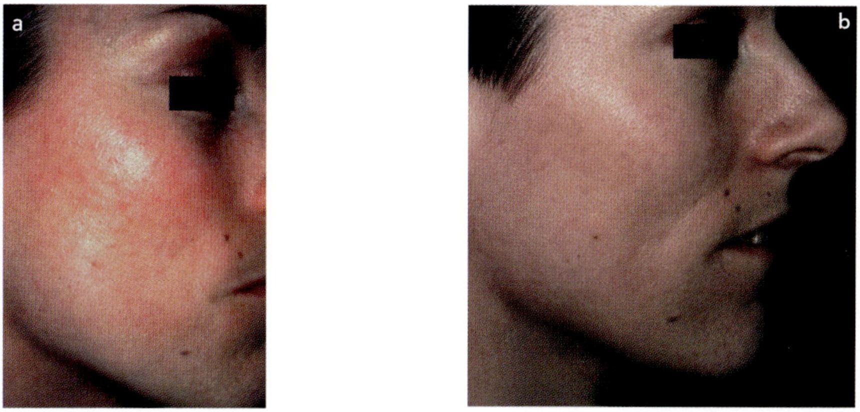

Figure 1 Superficial peel
Hyper-reactive skin with fine inflammatory folliculitis (a), after a superficial glycolic acid peel (b)
(photos J.-L. Vigneron)

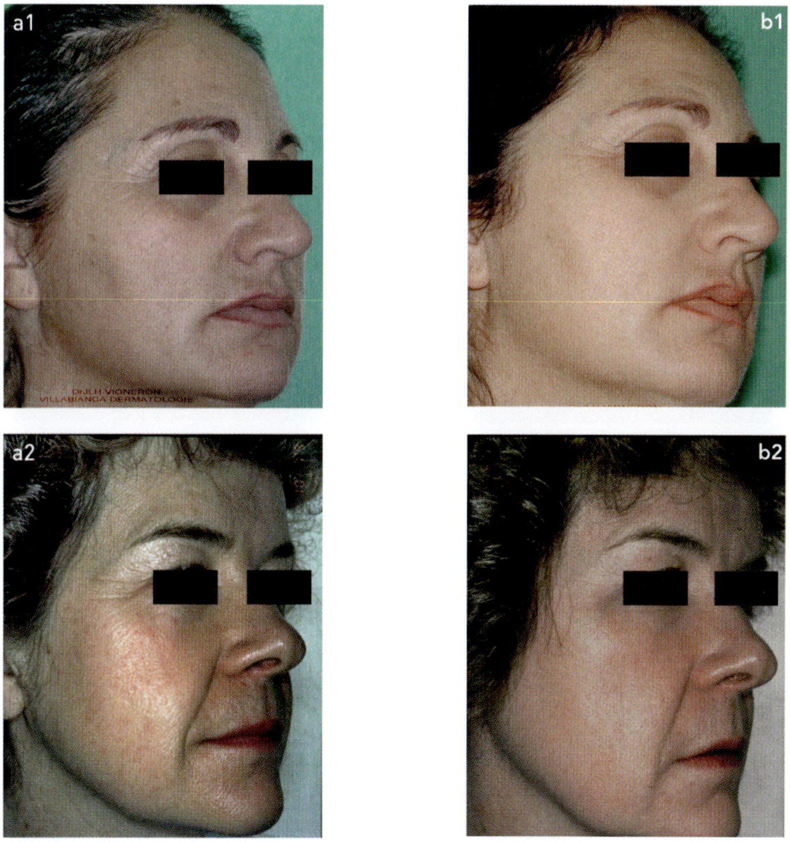

Figure 2 Medium 30% TCA peel
Mediterranean phototype. Dermatoheliosis 3 (a1), 6 weeks after 30% TCA peel (b1)
Caucasian phototype. Dermatoheliosis 3 (a2), 4 weeks after 30% TCA peel (b2)
(photos J.-L. Vigneron)

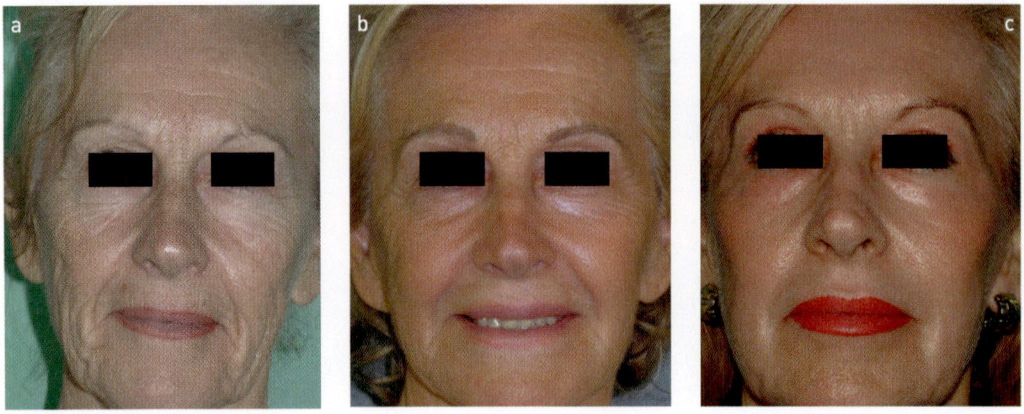

Figure 3 Exopeel deep peel
Age 68. Dermatoheliosis 4 (a), 2 months after Exopeel® (b), 11 years later, with no further treatments, age 79 (c). Note that the quality of the skin is much improved over its initial quality, 11 years earlier
(photos J.-L. Vigneron)

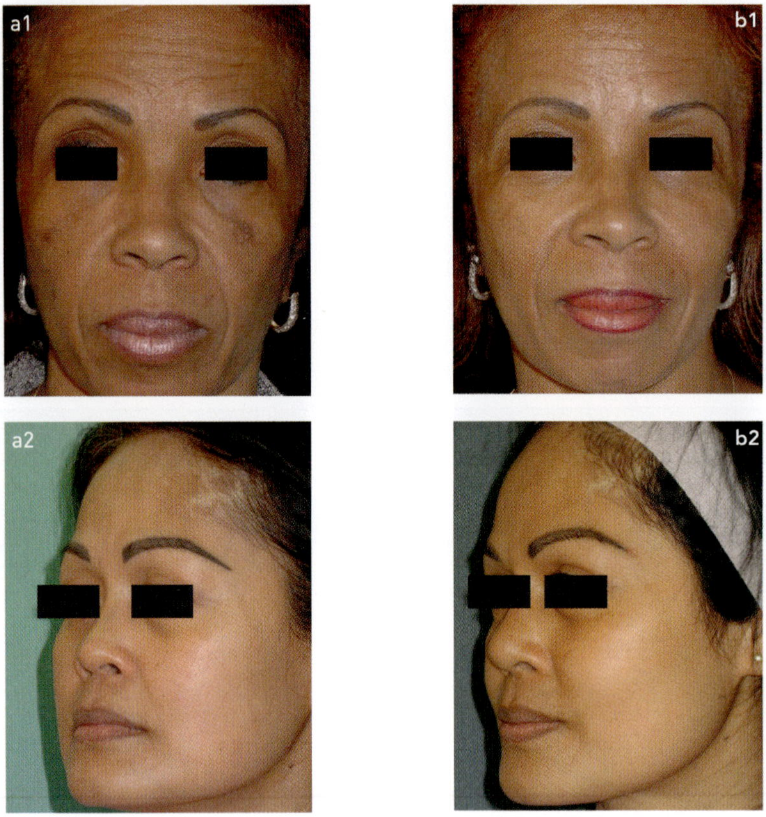

Figure 4 Specific spot peels
Caribbean phototype (a1), 2 months after SSP (SpotPeel®) (b1)
Thai phototype (a2), 6 months after SSP (SpotPeel®) (b2)
(photos J.-L. Vigneron)

Clinical case study: phenol peel Fig. 5

The results of phenol peels can surprise doctors as well as patients. This technique is highly standardised and the author has been carrying out this procedure since 1995 and then since 2005 under local anaesthetic only [3]. He has treated over 850 patients, and has trained numerous doctors in the technique. The results are reproducible, the recovery process can be predicted to the day, and the patient's experience is generally very good. It is the patient's family and friends who sometimes find themselves impressed.

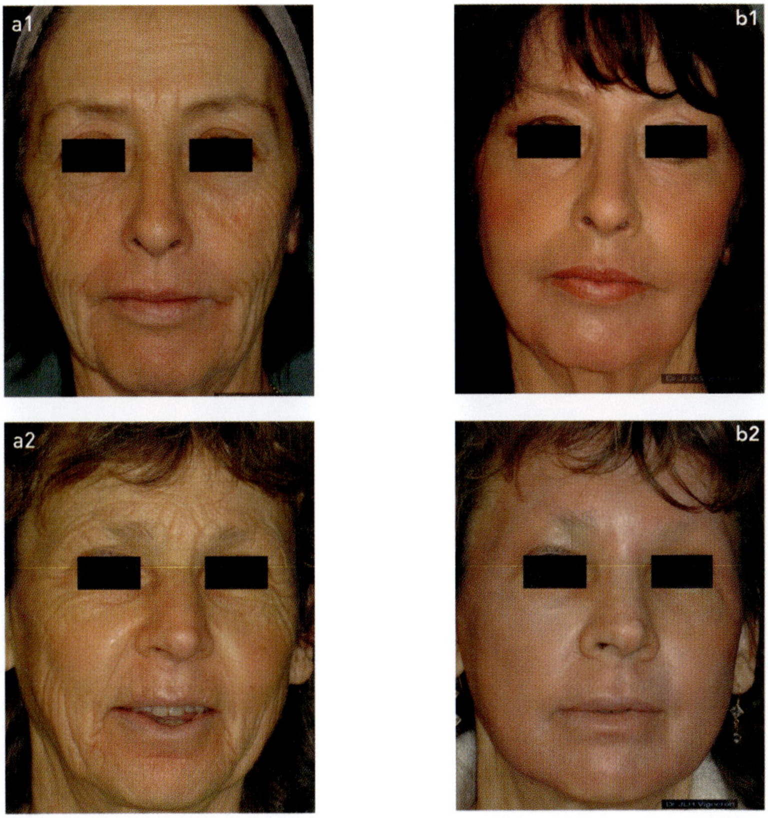

Figure 5 Phenol peel
Dermatoheliosis 4 + Ptosis (a1), 2 months after Exopeel®, phenol peel. The skin is smoother and the face is lifted. The cheeks are rounded, although they have not undergone any injections (b1)
Dermatoheliosis 4 + Ptosis (a2), 3 weeks after Exopeel®, the face is still pink but smooth and lifted (b2)
(photos J.-L. Vigneron)

It is important to emphasise that the results are sustainable. A second peel is required after around eleven years in the author's experience. Yet, after this 11-year period, wrinkles have only returned to the perioral and outer orbital regions (crows' feet), and the patient's wrinkles are never as important as they were before the first peel was performed. The extraordinary quality of the results over this period is the perfect illustration of the reverse effect as described by Butler [2].

This dermatological technique is underused by dermatologists.

MECHANICAL STIMULATION Fig. 6

Mechanical stimulation is a French technique based on Jacquet-Leroy pinch massage. Publications from 1907 and 1908 describe the simple pinching manœuvre that was initially proposed to treat acne. It consists of repeatedly applying pressure between the thumb and fingertip, as well as using the other fingers, thus targeting all depths of the skin and using all directions.

The manœuvre as put forward by Dr Jacquet (1907) was then taken up by Dr Leroy (1908) to treat acne and scarring.

For a long time, Jacquet-Leroy pinching has been considered to be the "massage of the stars" in France because of its effect on brightening the complexion and improving tone. One element of its success is that it is difficult to find a masseuse who is specialised in this technique.

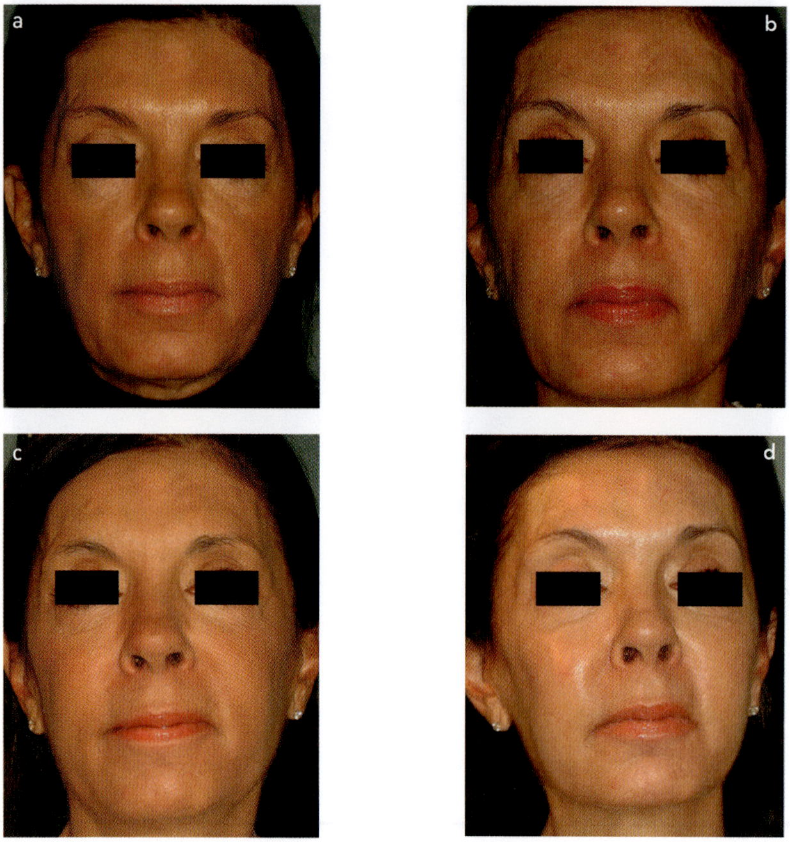

Figure 6 Mechanical stimulation
Weak facial outline (a), improved tone after 8 sessions of mechanical stimulation (b) and (c), Outcome after 7 months (d)
(photos J.-L. Vigneron)

Reproducing the manual treatment by machine

This is a medical device with a transducer that delivers microscopic pulses to the surface of the skin. Depending on the chosen pulse frequency and strength, the transducer generates different stimulations for specific aesthetic goals.

Scientific evidence

In one study, Revuz [4] showed a clinical improvement in firmness and facial shape. The same study also reported a histological change in skin structure in the treated area consisting in renewed dermal density due to an increase in collagen and elastin. Density was quantified in a later study and showed an increase of up to 240% in the best-case scenario.

In 2006 Varani [5] showed the effect of mechanical stimulation on fibroblast activity, with unexpectedly strong results. In addition, an action on endothelial cells, venous and lymphatic drainage, and improved adipocyte function was demonstrated (Max Lafontan) [6].

It can be drawn from all of these studies that a loss of mechanical tension seems to be the main factor explaining the fall in collagen synthesis in older skin [7].

For this reason the names mechanical stimulation and endermolift were put forward.

In a study yet to be published from Humbert, Jeudy, Fanian and Haftek, the following conclusions were made: in vitro tests demonstrated an 80.2% increase in hyaluronic acid, a 45.6% rise in elastin, a 7.8% increase in collagen type I, and a 115.4% rise in MMP9, together with fibroblasts showing an increased capacity for migration. Electron microscopy confirmed dermal remodelling correlated with signs of increased fibroblast activity in 50% of biopsies. A significant improvement in most of the clinical signs of aging was found. The patient satisfaction index (67% noted an improvement in skin laxity) was correlated with the improvement in the jowls (+ 25.52%).

The author's experience

We have been using this technique for two years. It has quickly found its place among the facial anti-aging treatments:

– either used alone to address facial shape, as a toner for the whole face and to soften and smooth scars;

– or in combination with other "minor interventions" with no visible aftermath: LED, LED-FOTOBoost™ aesthetic photodynamic therapy, superficial peels, or bipolar radiofrequency;

– or to prepare the skin for more aggressive interventions.

Conclusion: the new concept of "skin fitness"

It is important to capture trends. Today, Europe has yet to adopt a trend that is expanding rapidly in Asia known as skin fitness: it consists in regularly training and stimulating the skin through a combination of several techniques such as mechanical stimulation, superficial peels, and LED phototherapy, in the same way as other vital functions are maintained through a healthy lifestyle, nutrition, and physical exercise.

This gentle cellular stimulation is carried out regularly to maintain healthy and beautiful skin. Indeed, from the age of 25, fibroblast activity begins to diminish and the skin gradually loses elasticity, tone, and volume. The complexion turns yellow and grey very insidiously. By acting at the heart of the cells, LED, mechanical stimulation, peels, and new cosmetics are very effective methods to slow down the aging process. Combining them is synergistic.

CHEMICAL ADIPOCYTE LYSIS

For facial rejuvenation, this technique can be used to address the fat that builds up on the neck and chin over the years and widens the base of the face, a characteristic of age.

In the wake of adipocyte removal by aspiration through a cannula, a technique has been developed more recently that leads to adipocyte lysis through the injection of emulsifying substances.

There have been successive attempts to develop treatments to reduce localised deposits of adipose tissue or excess fat since the invention of liposuction around 1985 by Illouz and Fournier. In 1995 in the USA, Hoefflin used injections of a hypo-osmotic solution to break down adipocytes and in the same year in Sao Paolo, Patricia Rittes successfully injected phosphatidylcholine (PPC) into fatty pockets under the eyelids. In 2001, Franz Hasengschwandtner (Austria) defined the basic rules for the use of PPC in combination with deoxycholate (DOCA).

The technique of dissolving fat through PPC injections is called lipolysis.

What is lipolysis?

This treatment leads to the removal of stored fat in order to achieve a sculpting effect by non-surgical means. It is not a slimming treatment, nor is it the same as mesotherapy orhypo-osmolar lipotomy. It does not replace liposuction for the removal of large amount of fat.

Mode of action

Adipocytes are destroyed due to an action on the cell membrane. Adipocyte membranes are made of phospholipids with a hydrophilic and a hydrophobic part Fig. 7.

This hydrophobic-hydrophilic structure constitutes a double molecular layer, which is the basic structure of adipocyte membranes Fig. 8.

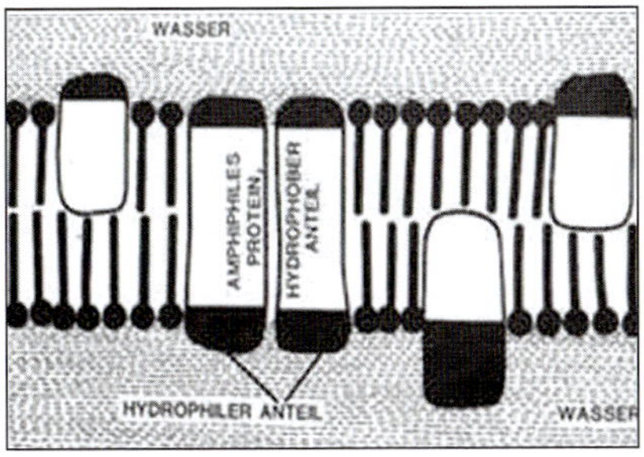

Figure 7 Cell membrane

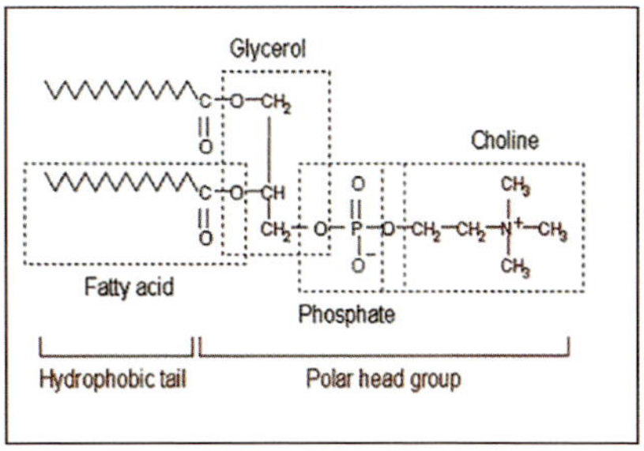

Figure 8 Basic hydrophobic-hydrophilic structure of cell membranes

Process of membrane destruction

The active molecules are: Phosphatidylcholine (a), Deoxycholate (b) and Benzyl alcohol (c) Fig. 9.

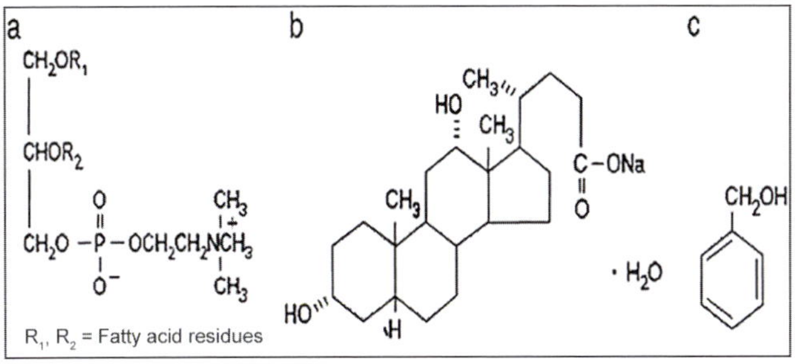

Figure 9 Active molecules (a-c)

The emulsification occurs due to the action of lipases: deoxycholate together with phosphatidylcholine emulsifies fat by causing a cascade of lipases to be released, which is required for membrane breakdown. The lipid particles push water back to the exterior. The fine fatty emulsion is dissolved by the lipases, and transported by HDL to the liver to be metabolised through beta-oxidation into the citric acid cycle Fig. 10.

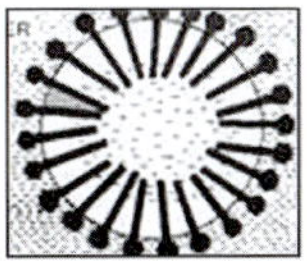

Figure 10 Lipid particle

In vivo mode of action

PPC causes adipocyte destruction through dephosphorylation. This is followed by an enzymatic cascade, and by the emulsification of fats that are transported to the liver, mainly by HDL. The metabolic products are then excreted by the intestines and kidneys in the form of fatty acids Fig. 11.

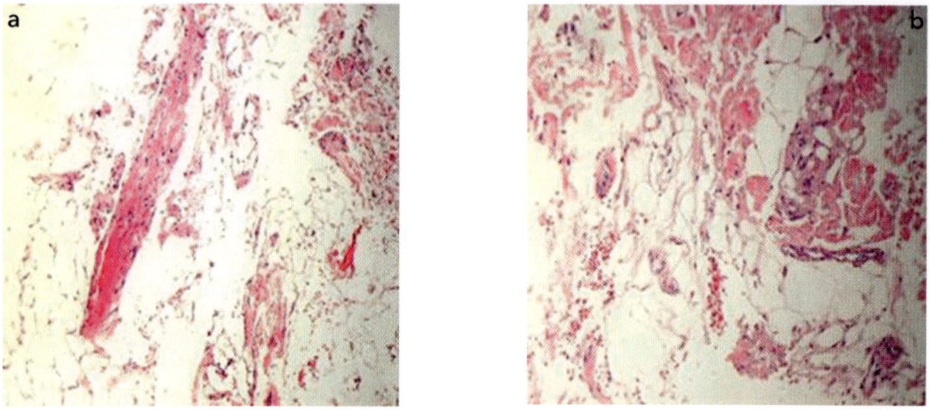

Figure 11 Histology: dissolution of adipocytes in vivo 10 days after lipolysis (a, b)
(Dr Hasengschwandtner – Austria)

Practising chemical lipolysis

Patient selection and information

The process begins by providing the patient with information and respecting the medical contra-indications: pregnant or breastfeeding women, diabetic patients with microvascular disease, and clotting disorders. The same is applicable to some auto-immune diseases (scleroderma, SLE, dermatomyositis, polymyositis), liver and kidney failure, some infectious diseases (tuberculosis, malaria, HIV), and finally any severe allergies or allergies to injected products.

A clinical examination determines the areas of the face where chemical lipolysis may be applied: jowls, double chin, and, according to some, the lower eyelids.

It is interesting to note that the preferred areas for chemical lipolysis are often those that are judged to be difficult or unsuitable for liposuction to treat.

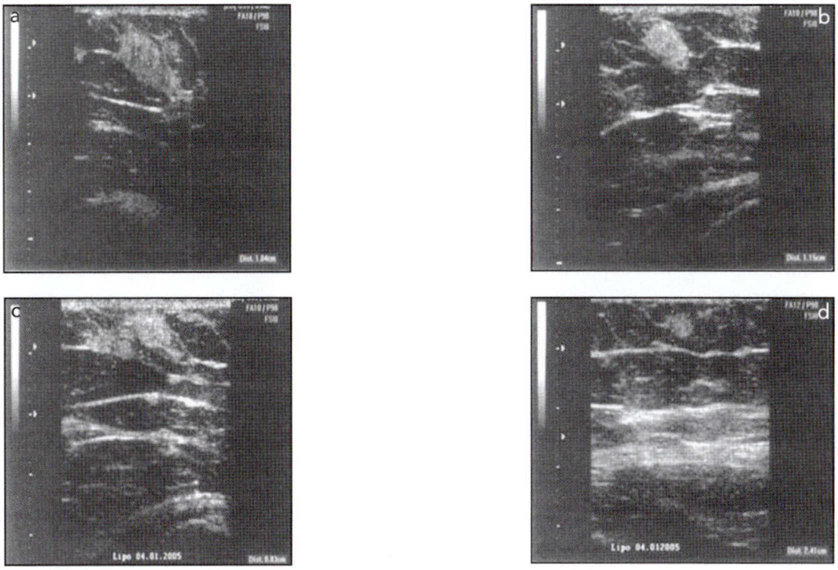

Figure 12 Sonography
Immediately after treatment (a), 4 weeks after treatment (b), 6 weeks after treatment (c), 8 weeks after treatment (d)
(Dr Norek – Austria)

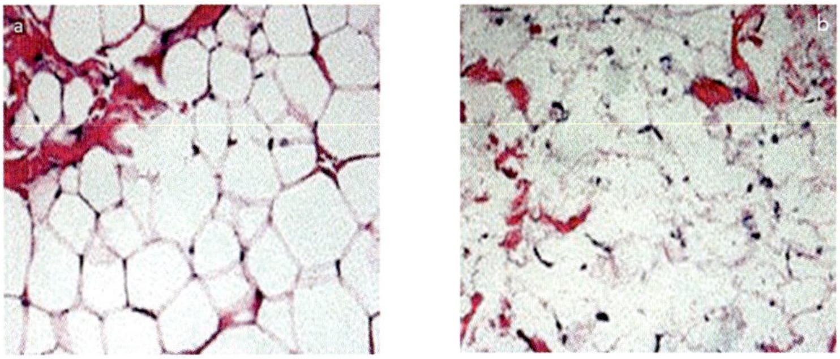

Figure 13 Histology: Adipocytes before (a) and after PPC treatment (b)
(University of California, Los Angeles, Dermatology Department, in vitro – Dermatol Surg 2004; 30: 1001-1008.)

Injection technique

After careful disinfection of the area to be treated, uniform subcutaneous (6-12 mm) injections are performed into the fat only. The choice of the formula and injection protocol must be very precise, respecting the maximum quantity to be injected in one session in order to avoid any excess concentration that could potentially cause necrosis.

Results with the approach that involves injecting large amount every six or eight weeks are markedly superior to those from treatment that consists in injections of small amount every two weeks.

In practical terms, to treat a small area of the jowls and a small amount of fat under the chin, prepare 8 ml of PPC solution added to 2 ml of xylocaine without adrenaline.

PPC acts over the course of more than eight weeks (gelatinous contact at four weeks), which means that there should be a one-month interval between sessions and a total of one or two sessions to treat the face.

Post-operative outcome

Oedema develops immediately along with pain, redness, and itching lasting between one and four days. After this the patient may experience some paraesthesia for two weeks. The following are reported from time to time: small temporary nodules, transient hyperpigmentation.

Side effects

Cases of anoxia of the tissue have been described, and in some cases this has led to necrosis. However, these cases have only involved treatment to the body and especially the internal surface of the thighs.

In all of these cases, the technique used deviated from standard procedures: too much product/palpable volume, injection depth was too superficial, or PPC was too concentrated.

The early warning signs are: intense redness in the treated area around a halo of vasoconstriction. The redness then develops into cyanosis. Preventive steps to take involve massaging deeply just after the injections.

Results

The author's experience covers 250 individuals, 50% of whom completed their treatment.

The cases are split evenly between those who had lipolysis carried out to the body and those whose face was treated.

The results of lipolysis procedures to the face are consistent, reproducible, and quick, with visible effects one month after the first session. We perform between one and three sessions Fig. 14 and 15.

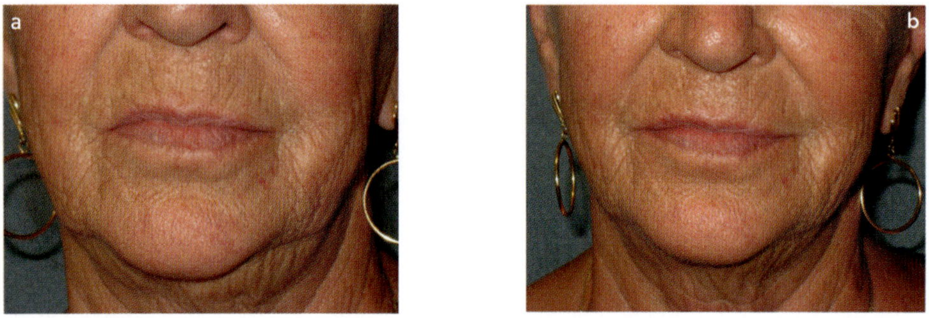

Figure 14 Chemical lipolysis
Excess adipose tissue in an elastic skin (a). After chemical lipolysis. Effective result despite an elastic skin (b) *(photos J.-L. Vigneron)*

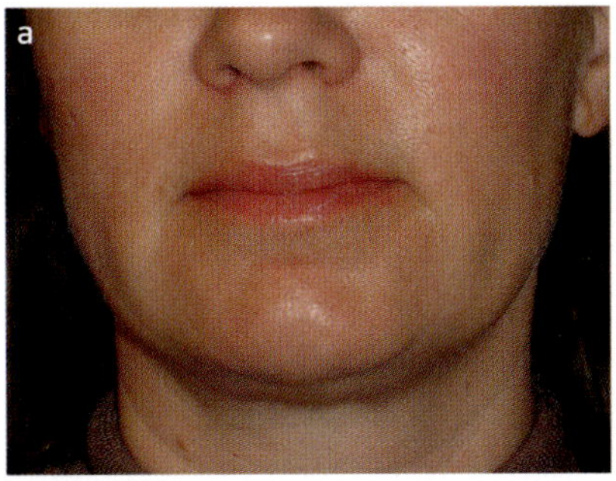

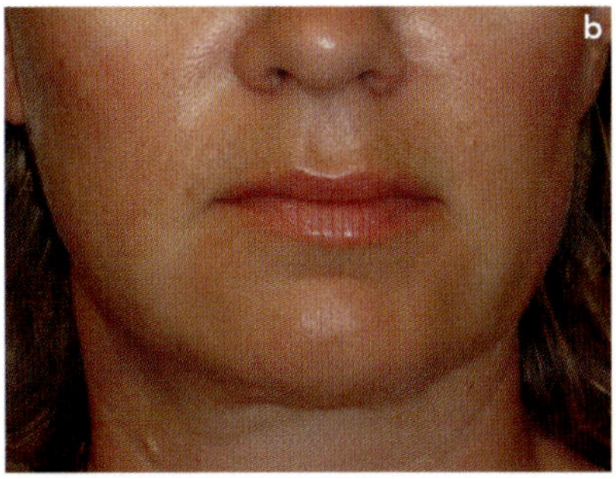

Figure 15 Chemical lipolysis
Excess adipose tissue in the jowls (a). Bulk removed from the lower face by chemical lipolysis (b) *(photos J.-L. Vigneron)*

Legislation

Since 2011, chemical lipolysis has been banned in France. The reasons remain unclear, because the age of the method and the tens of thousands of cases treated suggest that the technique should remain in use. At the same time when the sudden decision to ban this treatment was made, a study on the method was permitted to continue. This study will soon lead to the product being returned to the market.

Table 2 Can chemical lipolysis compete with liposuction?

	Liposuction	Lipolysis
Psychological impact	Fear of GA Morbidity related to hospital admission	Better perception of this method No serious incident
Around the intervention	Detachment of deeper planes Local or regional haematomas Long and obligatory period of immobilisation Risk of proximal oedema Risk of asymmetry	No detachment Local subcutaneous haematomas No immobilisation Oedema very rare after 5 days Corrects asymmetry
Result on surface appearance	Minimal action on skin quality Skin can remain flabby and distended Risk of a dimpled texture	Action on skin quality Skin has renewed tightness and firmness Renewed smoothness
Results for the patient	Immediate result Fat is removed in one session Widespread and deep areas treated Satisfaction ++ (Statistics?)	Results are gradual over 2-6 months ~ 30% less fat per session Small and medium depth areas treated Satisfaction measured after full course of treatment: – very satisfied 65% – satisfied 18% – mediocre 10% – failed 7% (university research following patients between 2003 and 2005 taking 8,000 treatments into account)

The author thanks Network Lipolysis, Dr Franz Hasengschwandtner and Dirk Brandl for their technical and scientific support.

THREAD LIFT

This treatment originated in Korea. Obtaining good results using simple techniques with a straightforward recovery is the dream of patients, doctors, and insurers! The thread lift with short threads or V-Lift is one of these techniques.

Material

The procedure uses threads made from PDS (polydioxanone), which are absorbable. The thread is mounted in a needle. Along the length of the needle, it is held externally by a sliding clip.

A 6/0 thread in a 29G needle is used to treat the face.

There are two needle lengths available: 25 mm and 38 mm needles are used with 30 mm and 60 mm threads respectively Fig. 16.

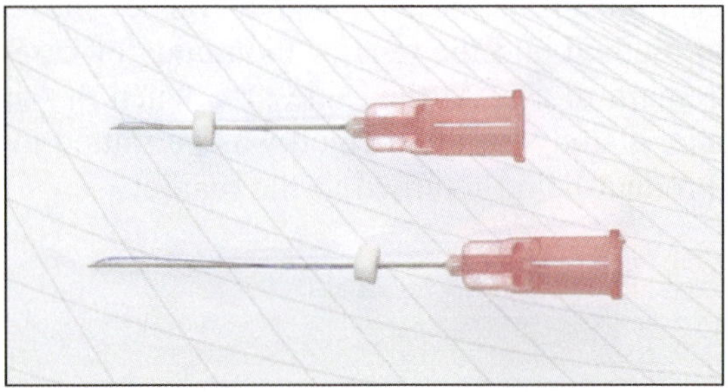

Figure 16 25 mm and 38 mm needles

Method

The skin is cleaned. Anaesthesia is not required. The short threads are placed in situ one by one, alongside each other, to form a relatively dense mesh Fig. 17.

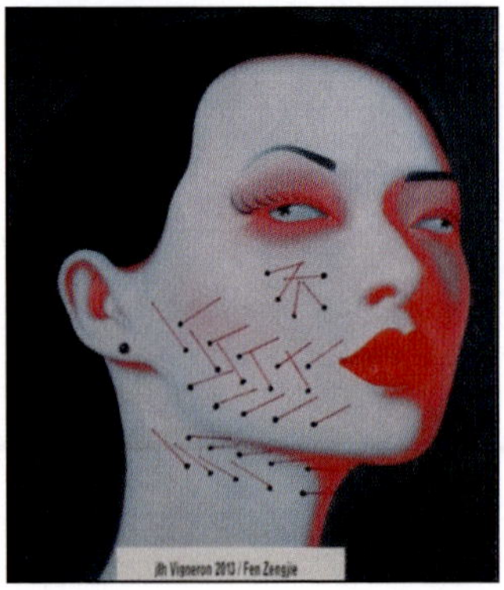

Figure 17 Short threads on a Fen Zengjie drawing

The patient must be lying down or even in the Trendelenburg position so that the facial tissues at rest are uplifted. The needle must be inserted in one movement, without hesitation or any withdrawal, so that the thread can be correctly positioned. The practitioner tries to arrange the thread directions to cross over from one row to the next. Working quickly and confidently makes anaesthesia superfluous.

Number: 20-25 60 mm threads per cheek, 15 in the area under the jawline, and ten 30 mm threads for the midline under the chin. More can be added lower down the neck Fig. 18.

One session of this kind is carried out, followed by a second 4-6 weeks later, with half or a third of the total number of threads.

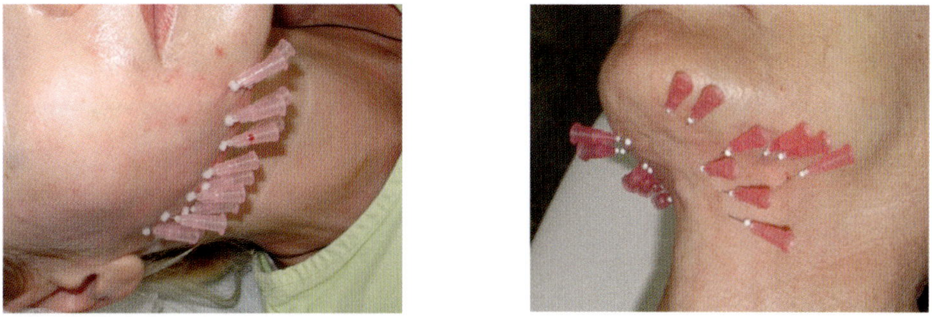

Figure 18 Needles in situ (thread lift)
(photos J.-L. Vigneron)

Results

What results can be expected with the use of these smooth threads, which are so short and thin? Fig. 19 and 20

No lifting effect is achieved, such as what can be seen in a correctly performed treatment using many very long, barbed threads that are then pulled taut. It should be noted that this type of intervention has a longer recovery.

There are two types of improvement:

– the mesh formed by more than 60 threads inserted in one session in a horizontal or tilted position restores the outline with an action on facial shape;

– the number of threads placed in the dermis and subcutaneous tissue creates a fine layer of collagen. The result is a softening of the contours, and small shadows disappear.

In fact the result is the same as what would be obtained with a filler if it could be spread in a very fine layer very evenly over a very large surface, with in addition a mild renewed skin-tightening or lifting effect.

Patients are very happy with these results and the satisfaction index is very high, which is always surprising and gratifying when such a gentle technique is used.

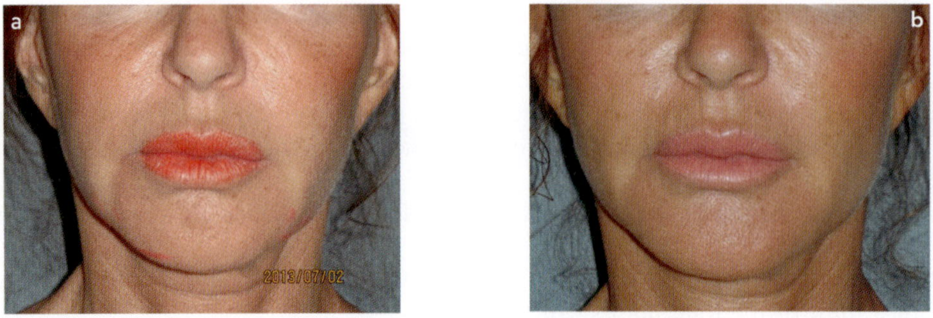

Figure 19 Results of a thread lift with short threads
Before treatment (a), after intervention (b)
(photos J.-L. Vigneron)

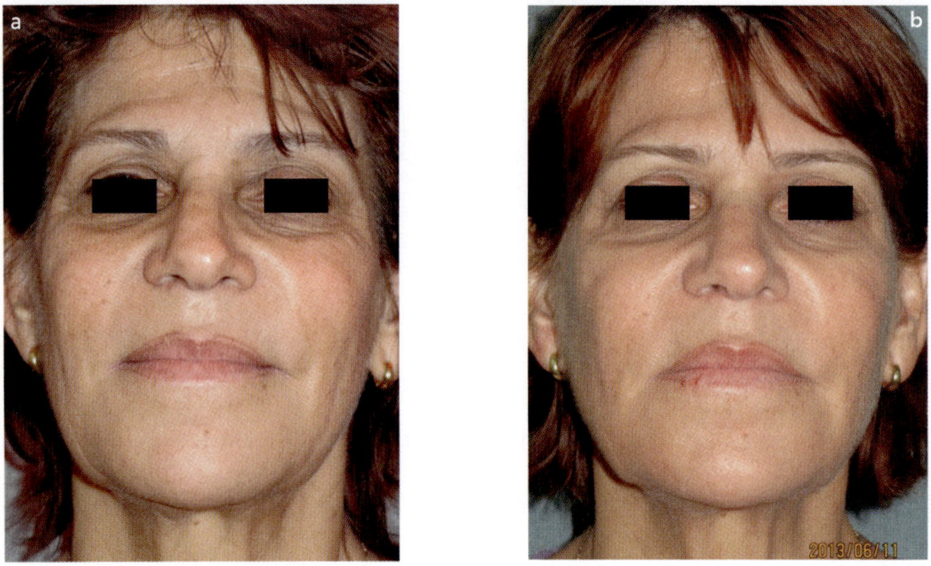

Figure 20 Results of a thread lift with short threads
Before treatment (a), after intervention (b)
(photos J.-L. Vigneron)

Conclusion

Thread lifting with short threads is a new technique that softens the facial contours and offers a mild lifting effect. The cheeks, facial outline, and neck are the best areas for treatment. No other technique that is so straightforward to achieve offers this type of effect. The results are subtle but clear and patients' expectations are met.

REFERENCES

[1] Stegman SJ. A study of dermabrasion and chemical peels in an animal model. J Dermatol Surg Oncol 1980; 6: 490-497.
[2] Butler Peter EM, *et al.* Quantitative and qualitative effects of chemical peeling on photo-aged skin: an experimental study. Plast Reconstr Surg 2001; 107: 222.
[3] Vigneron J.-L. Peeling profond phénolé, la révolution anesthésique. GRCD 2006; 39: 01.
[4] Revuz J, Adhoute H, Cesarini JP, Poli F, Lacarriere C, Emiliozzi C. Clinical and histological effects of the Lift6® device used on facial skin aging. Nouv Dermatol 2002; 21: 335-342.
[5] Varani J, Dame Mk, Rittie L, Fligiel Se, Kang S, Fisher Gj, Voorhees JJ. Decreased collagen production in chronologically aged skin: roles of age-dependent alteration in fibroblast function and defective mechanical stimulation. Am J Pathol 2006 Jun; 168(6): 1861-1868.
[6] Marques Ma, Combes M, Roussel B, Vidal-Dupont L, Thalamas C, Lafontan M, Viguerie N. Impact of a mechanical massage on gene expression profile and lipid mobilization in female gluteofemoral adipose tissue. Obes Facts 2011; 4(2): 121-129.
[7] Shoham N, Gefen A. Mechanotransduction in adipocytes. J Biomech 2012 Jan; 45(1): 1-8.

CHAPTER 11

Laser treatment consultation

Bertrand Pusel

INTRODUCTION

The number of procedures carried out worldwide to manage facial skin aging is always on the increase as a result of the ever-expanding development of new technologies for this indication, and because of increased demand of patients seeking to look younger, a trend that has been broadly spread by the media.

While treatments using lasers or related technologies, such as radiofrequency or ultrasound, are aesthetic procedures, they remain wholly within the sphere of medical interventions so they are subject to a "best endeavours" obligation and a requirement to provide patient information.

In addition, in an aesthetic context, when the procedure is not required out of therapeutic necessity, the obligation to proceed with best endeavours is considered stronger than ever.

This means that the consultation prior to treatment is of crucial importance and it must allow the patient to obtain clear, full, and honest information.

It also considers the patient holistically, taking both body and mind into account when it comes to their request, the possible consequences of the treatment, and the results achieved.

The consultation does not simply consist of a description of the procedure, but it encompasses how the procedure is monitored. This requires a significant investment from the doctor's part.

It ends with the patient being given an information letter and consent form.

This means that the practitioner is subject to a three-pronged medical liability: civil liability, criminal liability, and disciplinary action, as well as being obliged to respect professional confidentiality.

PRIOR CONSULTATION

The patient's request

The patient's request needs to be suitably clarified, so that the procedure offered provides the best possible fit, and this means that the practitioner will need to spend time listening attentively to the patient.

The general and non-specific expression "facial aging", for example, is often used and it could correspond to wide-ranging clinical realities depending on whether patients are concerned about their solar lentigines, perioral wrinkles, or erythema and telangiectasias, each of which requires a specific treatment. It is also important to gain an understanding of the patient's psychological motivation for taking these steps: whether they have personal, family (e.g. divorce) or professional reasons (looking for employment, physical appearance unrelated to that required for their job, etc.).

Medical history

The interview needs to be carried out meticulously. Patient's age, lifestyle and habits will be discussed: exposure to the sun with or without photoprotection, tobacco use, alcohol consumption, hormonal status, and skin care routine.

The patient's medical history must be detailed to identify any autoimmune disease, previous surgical interventions (quality of healing), recurrent herpes, contact allergy or dermatitis, dermatological disorder that could be exacerbated through the Koebner phenomenon, and current or previous medications (oral isotretinoin, corticosteroids, hormone replacement therapy in females).

Clinical examination

It is crucial to ascertain the patient's exact phototype. This will state the indication and follow-up for some treatments as well as the risk of complications, especially in terms of pigmentation and scarring.

The lesions for treatment must be assessed correctly: type, extent, location (any risk of keloid scarring), and quality of adjacent integumentary system structures.

A full examination must be undertaken to investigate whether there are any other lesions to be treated (lentigines, erythrosis interfollicularis colli, etc.) or dermatological abnormalities meaning extra care will need to be taken while carrying out the treatment (psoriasis, vitiligo, etc.).

Understanding psychological factors

The psychological impact of the lesions to be treated must also be taken into account. It is essential to assess the patient from a psychological point of view in order to ensure that the procedure is being carried out under the right conditions.

In particular, the history will look for any previous aesthetic procedures that have already been performed, their result, and the patient's satisfaction with them. It is important to understand how to identify patients whose wishes are unrealistic, especially in body dysmorphic disorder, or major psychological disorders such as severe depression.

Studies have shown that these kinds of patients frequently seek and undergo aesthetic procedures.

Patient information and informed consent

The purpose of the laser treatment consultation is to describe realistic results, how the procedure and the post-operative follow-up are carried out, and to set out the risks, while establishing a trusting relationship.

Consent can only be obtained when the patient has received clear, genuine, appropriate and intelligible information.

More generally, a laser treatment consultation must prioritise a good understanding of the treatment protocol and the risks it entails, the expected results, and compliance with the requirements of post-operative care.

Only a doctor can present this information and it must be tailored to the patient. Although the patient is given a written document, under no circumstances does this mean the doctor can dispense with the oral explanation, or view the written document as a substitute.

The description of the procedure must be part of the oral explanation: the benefit patient can expect to see (duration, anticipated number of sessions, the need for maintenance treatments, etc.) the conditions of the intervention (type of anaesthesia if any, level of pain to be expected, etc.), post-operative outcome, normal recovery period, precautions to be taken with regard to exposure to the sun, whether they need to be accompanied home or will be unable to drive a car, and the aftercare as well as any potential complications of the procedure.

The written consent does not summarise the patient information and it only confirms the various aspects that make up the process of providing patient information.

Moreover, information should be specific to each technology applied and must not attempt to cover all procedures.

Additional information forms to be given to the patient are useful but they must, whenever possible, be validated by relevant bodies and regularly updated in view of new data from the literature. Informed consent implies that the doctor is bound to clearly present to the patient all the risks of the procedure under consideration that can reasonably be predicted in view of current scientific knowledge and the consequences that these could entail, and the physician should be confident that the patient has understood the various aspects.

Once this information has been provided, both written and spoken, the patient must have realistic expectations of the treatment's results and risks, allowing them to make a fully informed decision.

Finally, it is useful to give the patient preoperative recommendations and a prescription for any aftercare that is needed during the recovery period.

In some countries, it has even been suggested that a non-guarantee clause should be included to warn the patient that although the technique used may be effective in the majority of cases, there can be no guarantee on an individual basis or in their specific case.

Quote

In some countries, it is mandatory to provide a quote for aesthetic procedures that is more than just an estimated sum or one that is provided only on patient request.

In France, for example, the quote must be provided 15 days prior to the procedure. This period can be reduced to seven days if the patient expressly requests it in writing. Observation of this process would doubtless be subject to close consideration in the event of a complication giving rise to legal proceedings.

Making photographic records

Photos are essential and must be taken as a matter of course so that the patient's condition before treatment can be compared to that after treatment, and the results assessed.

In fact they constitute medico-legal documents with no substitute that will be requested in the event of any litigation being brought forward.

Particular attention must be paid to who owns the rights to the image in view of any potential use of photographic records for either scientific or commercial purposes. It is highly recommended that the patients are asked for their authorisations specifying any limitations for the use of photographs.

Pre-treatment test

It is not essential to perform a laser test in the majority of indications but it can have a number of uses.

– It reassures the patient in terms of how the procedure will unfold and the efficacy of the technique.

– It allows the doctor to determine the optimum treatment parameters.

– It allows the doctor to ensure that there will be no complications, especially in terms of pigmentation for subjects with dark phototypes.

– It is useful for medico-legal purposes.

It must, for all of the reasons above, be carried out prior to treatment whenever warranted in view of the type of intervention and the patient's case.

TREATMENT

This is when the laser treatment consultation becomes a reality and the process must involve recording information about the patient and the procedure being carried out with the same level of rigour as would apply to medical notes as they will have a significant legal value in the event of a complaint.

Some types of intervention may be carried out under local or general anaesthesia, which means that a hospital admission may potentially be required.

Prior to laser treatment, it is therefore advisable to draw up a proper "pre-operative" check-list that reiterates all the essentials of the pre-operative consultation: checking that the patient is fully informed, collecting a quote where necessary, taking pre-operative photographs, ensuring compliance with recommendations and treatments prescribed (for example applying anaesthetic cream, herpes prevention starting the day before treatment).

At this stage, it must be stated that laser treatments or treatments using related techniques must not be performed if they fall outside the doctor's sphere of competence or if the doctor has not undergone appropriate training.

In addition, it is crucial that only validated treatments should be performed, in accordance with the data from scientific studies.

Furthermore, the doctor must have the necessary means available and must practice in a suitable environment so that the patient is not exposed to unnecessary risks.

The treatments must take place:

- in a room that has been made available for this purpose;
- under clean and aseptic conditions;
- following the rules of good practice for each of the technologies used.

At the end of the treatment, the doctor must remain available to explain what the post-operative recommendations are, as well as the precautions to be taken with regard to exposure to the sun. A prescription will be given to the patient for the products required along with a description of how they should be used depending on the treatment carried out.

POST-TREATMENT CONSULTATION

Following treatment with lasers or related technologies, a post-operative consultation is not necessarily carried out as a matter of course but it is always advisable in order to relieve patient anxiety.

However, there are some circumstances in which it is essential:

- if the laser intervention breaks down the epidermis, as is the case with all ablative techniques, whether fractional or conventional. Early and repeated post-operative follow-up is essential to detect and diagnose any predictive complications and to medically manage them;
- in cases when there are risks related to the patient, such as the management of inflammatory hyper-pigmentation in subjects with high phototypes;
- when it is useful to evaluate the results by taking photos for either scientific or medico-legal purposes.

As is the case after any therapeutic intervention, the doctor must be available to the patient to offer the best management of any complications, but also to assist with post-operative stress. While the patient may understand that a complication could arise, they will not in any way accept a lack of availability on the part of their doctor and if this happened, it would of course be likely to lead to a major crisis in the doctor-patient relationship causing legal proceedings when they could be avoided.

It is advisable to give the patients a telephone number on which they can reach the doctor at any time if post-operative problems occur.

In the event of a serious complication, patients should not hesitate to contact a doctor's civil and professional liability insurance provider.

CONCLUSION

As with any medical intervention, treatments using lasers or related technologies involve an overall management of the patient, without omitting the psychological aspect. It is particularly important to focus on providing the patient with good quality information and ensure that they have fully understood, meaning that they are able to give their free and informed consent.

This is a real prerequisite for optimising the results of treatment: to set out clearly and in a trustworthy manner the possible complications and to avoid disappointing the patient by exaggerating potential results, as these could both be a potential source of conflict.

The availability of the practitioner before, during, and after the laser treatment, together with their listening skills, are the natural counterparts to a good quality prior training.

REFERENCES

[1] Evenou P. Prise en charge globale du vieillissement cutané: indications respectives de la cosmétologie et des différentes techniques. Encycl Med Chir (Cosmétologie et dermatologie esthétiques) 2000; 50-490, A 10: 5 p.

[2] Goldberg D. Legal considerations in cosmetic laser surgery. J Cosmet Dermatol 2006; 5(2): 103-106.

[3] Greve B, Raulin C. Professionnal errors cause by lasers and Intense Pulsed Light Technology in Dermatology and aesthetic medicine, preventive strategies and case studies. Dermatol Surg 2002; 28(2): 151-161.

[4] Horton S, Alster ST. Preoperative and postoperative considerations for carbon dioxide laser resurfacing. Cutis 1999; 64: 399-406.

[5] Mc Burney E. Side effects and complications of laser therapy. Dermatol Clinics 2002; 20: 165-176.

CHAPTER 12

Lasers and related technologies, combined treatments in medical and cosmetic surgery

Benjamin Ascher

INTRODUCTION

Whatever the morphological type of the face may be, most of the time and for any type of aging, expression lines are always associated to aging: muscle ptosis, fat, and skin sagging are treated by lifting; lipoatrophy is treated by filler or lipofillings; excess fat is treated by liposuccion. Any surface alteration is to be treated by laser, ultrasound, radiofrequency and associated techniques, as well as abrasive methods such as peeling.

Lasers, botulinum toxin injections and fillers are not meant to replace upper, mid, or lower face and neck lifts; on the contrary, they are often combined with these procedures and optimize their result [1-3]. This combination of medical and surgical treatments is one of the main current trends in plastic surgery and cosmetic dermatology.

LASERS AND RELATED TECHNOLOGIES ASSOCIATED TO INJECTIONS

Wrinkles and other spots which are mainly located near the lower eyelids and the cheeks, as well as near the periorbital and circumoral areas, cannot be entirely treated with either intradermal or subcutaneous injections.

Lasers are desirable at the surface, either by producing an epidermal ablation on a continuous or fractionated mode, or by producing a dermal stimulation by "heating", or both. Please note that this dermal stimulation adds to the different stimulations caused by injections, such as mechanical (cutting needle, cannula) injections, physicochemical injections of fillers, or biological injections with lipofilling. This stimulation also adds to dermal stimulation, which is constantly observed in the areas that have been discolored during a lift. Surgical dissection has produced a mechanical stimulation of the superficial dermis [4-10].

What procedure should we start with?

This is still debated through publications: lasers can precede or follow injections. However, they should not be associated or used at the same time, since the hyaluronic acid, other fillers and fat cells (especially during superficial injections) can have their properties denaturalized by the "laser heating" and can eventually produce side effects, such as oedemas, inflammatory reactions and even infections. This applies in the case of the CO_2 laser and the hyaluronic acid in histological analysis, and to a lesser extent in clinical studies. However, the Yag, IPL and RF do not seem to generate any effect [11-13] and the lasers do not seem to denaturalize toxins [14-16].

Botulinum toxin appears to have an increasing preparation use for lasers or filler injections. Muscle relaxation, which is produced when botulinum toxin is injected or following another medical procedure, appears to be a way to optimize and then to extend the results. It must not be injected during another ongoing medical or surgical treatment in order to avoid its diffusion to other muscles through the edema resulting from this treatment. Most authors consider that the toxin can be diffused at up to 2 cm, but it has been shown that its diffusion capacity exceeds 3 cm, particularly in the case of injections of large volumes or bleedings [17, 18]. This is the reason why we recommend that the injected volume should range between 0.05 and 0.1 cm^3 per injection point.

Act step by step with a treatment planning

It's a true revolution within our practice, which started a few years ago following two main axes:

– treatments are medical before anything: until the 1990s, patients would leave it to the almighty surgeon, sole chief on board, who was the one deciding to go with a heavy procedure. The surgical act was admittedly disabling but "miraculous" and supposed to resolve anything, although it required the patient to stop working sometimes during several weeks.

As of today, much has changed: results have to be optimum without causing the patient any pain and without forcing him/her to get on sick leave. First, we perform an active medical act, yet as minimally invasive as possible. It's a natural evolution followed by the whole medicine practice, and botulinum toxin injections are one of the main illustrations of that trend within the aesthetic surgery segment. Second, when for a single problem there is a medical and a surgical treatment option, the medical option is chosen, even if it has to shake our surgeons' ego. It must also be noted that we actually integrated the best medical techniques within our practice for a while;

– medical or surgical treatment has to be a part of a plan and of a protocol. We now treat step by step: it guarantees more discreet and longer-lasting results. If the first surgical or medical treatment is a success, it can be maintained by regular but delayed complementary treatments, active but non invasive. The botulinum toxin is the perfect illustration of that planning method.

LASERS AND INJECTIONS ASSOCIATED WITH EYELID SURGERY

If cosmetic indications prevent the upper eyelid to get toxin injections, the lower eyelid is often treated this way, in accordance with the crow's feet indications.

What is the best interval between the injection of botulinum toxin and the surgical procedure? Although there is no global consensus [1], a minimum of 15 days [2, 19], or, even better, 3 weeks before surgery and 1 to 2 months after [20, 21], seems to be reasonable.

Toxin and eyelid

The resulting immobilization of the orbicularis, a wide and powerful depressor muscle, has multiple advantages.

– **Before:** minimum 3 weeks before lower eyelid blepharoplasty: whether transconjunctival or subciliary, it helps to treat crow's feet, which surgery does not correct, and reduces traction on scar tissue, ectropion, and transient conjunctivitis. Diminishing tension of the skin and muscles reduces tension on the stitches and operated areas, and may improve the healing as well as scarring processes[1]. However, this preparatory treatment has two disadvantages: a greater risk of oedema due to lack of massage of the eyelid lymph vessels, and difficulties in outlining the skin to be excised before the surgery, if the patient has not been photographed before the injection.

– **After:** between 1 and 6 months after lower eyelid blepharoplasty: botulinum toxin injections reduce any residual hypertonia in the orbicularis, as well as surface lines. These lines must be treated with microdoses (1-2 points of 1 unit of Botox®/Vistabel®, 1-2 unit of Xeomin®/Bocouture® or 2,5-5 units of Dysport®/Azzalure®), especially in the infero and external lateral area of the eyelid [22-27].

Laser and eyelid

We shall not insist on the remarquable breakthrough of lower eyelid surgery by transconjunctival incision with CO_2 laser, allowing a very precise exeresis of fat hernias causing fat pockets. The electrical bistoury allows that operation but with less precision [3, 28, 29] Fig. 1.

The resurfacing laser, especially of the lower eyelid, complements this transconjunctival blepharoplasty and allows to avoid skin ablation, which is a lot less necessary than what the patients think, thus avoiding round eyes and ectropions. But this continuous or

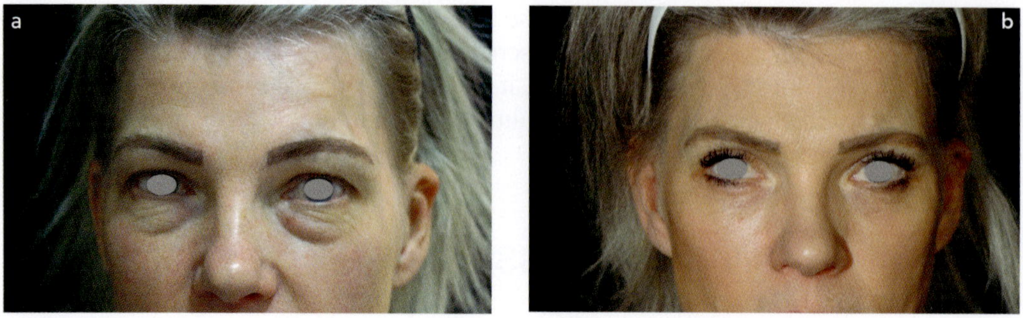

Figure 1 Blepharoplasty on 4 eyelids. On the lower eyelid, comination of resurfacing CO_2 laser and Erbium with a laser CO_2 transconjunctival blepharoplasty. (a) Before treatment, result after 3 years (b)

fractionated resurfacing with CO_2, whether it is associated with Erbium Yag or not (like on the Derma k® mode), can be used on its own in the case of superficial wrinkles without any other age spots. With constants that are adapted to the eyelids, its results are often positive, lasting and better than chemical peeling. The botulinum toxin injection, when performed 3 weeks prior to this resurfacing (as prior to injections of hyaluronic acid), can improve wound healing and optimize the result by reducing muscle contractions. After the procedure, the duration of redness can be reduced to 10-15 days by applying a Lumiderm type healing bandage for 4 days, an ophthalmic Dexamethasone ointment for 7 days (Sterdex type), as well as a healing ointments (like "eye contours"). Of course, sun protection must be respected in order to avoid dark spots that follow redness. In case of recurrent wrinkles, this resurfacing can be repeated 6 months to 1 year later.

LASERS AND INJECTIONS ASSOCIATED WITH FACELIFTS

The lifting of ptosed deep tissues (fat and muscles) can only be performed by surgical intervention, either without dissection or detachment, the result of which has a limited duration (approximately 2 years), or with a certainly more invasive method (although a lot less invasive than ten years ago), which lasts for approximately 10 years, which involves lifting techniques.

Upper face

The toxin-surgery association is a must when treating the upper face.

However, when the relaxation of the forehead and the eyebrows is major, and when the periorbital and zygomatic areas must also be lifted, the associated use of the toxin with the surgical treatment should be preferred. When injected prior to a facelift, especially in the upper-lateral (temporal-zygomatic) region, and in case of detachment of the middle third of the face, botulinum toxin considerably reduces the operation duration (since there is no muscle section), post-surgical healing and side-effects (alopecia, residual pain, wound healing, flattened areas). It contributes to the optimization of inadequate surgical results, either performed immediately or at a later stage, by correcting residual asymmetries or post-surgical facial paralysis, which is often transient, but can also persist in a long term [20, 21-33]. Horizontal lines located on the forehead are generally better treated with botulinum toxin than with surgery.

To avoid that the depressor muscles, mainly the external part of the orbicularis, pull down the tissues and decrease or even erase the lifting short-terms results, it is interesting to inject botulinum toxin into the forehead muscle and the crows' feet muscle in order to prepare the surgery. The external orbicular, the muscle surrounding the eye, is the most harmful and has to be neutralized in priority. That preparation, whose outcome is a muscular immobilization before surgery, improves the scaring process and the lifting results post-surgery. A couple of years later, regular botulinum toxin injections will prolong the lifting results. Eventually, in most cases, there is no real interest to perform a second lifting 10 or 20 years later. Indeed, the toxin (combined with hyaluronic acids, peelings or lasers) avoids a second course of surgery.

Alongiside toxine, abrasions by peeling or laser treat surface lines and heliodermis stigmas, and by the "tensing" effect [34] they create in the dermoepidermic region, they complete on the surface what the lifting has created in depth. Recently, the tensing effect on the forehead by focalised ultrasounds has been mentioned but only clinical studies may allow a conclusion. The fillers, mainly of hyaluronic acid, help treat the fine lines and harmonize the missing volumes by completing the lifting, especially around the eyebrow and the upper eyelid Fig. 2.

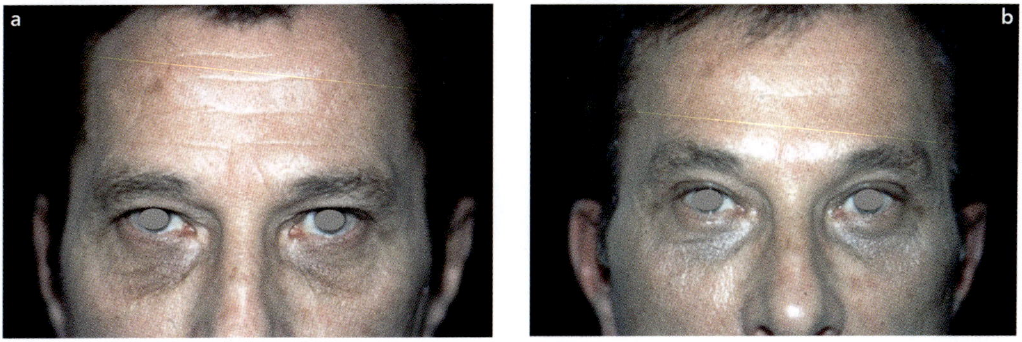

Figure 2 Lifting of the upper third of the face by small scars on the forehead and blepharoplasty on 4 eyelids by laser CO_2 laser
(a) Before operation, result after 5 years (b)

Mid- or lower third of the face

Volumators, either exogenous (hyaluronic acid and equivalents) or endogenous (fat), treat the lack of volumes that lifting can not heal: lipofilling is part of the modern lifting, and it avoids the detachment of tissues by lifting on these lipoatrophic regions [35].

On surface, lasers, in their ablative and non-ablative mode, besides heliodermis treatment, can create a non-negligible tensing effect, even though it is limited in time. They are often used during lifting on areas that can not be treated by lifting: around the perilabial and the lower eyelid, mostly to treat dermoepidermic lines. However, resurfacing is less and less used on the areas that have just been detached by a lifting, due to the high risk of necrosis. It remains an effective treatment, especially in its non-ablative mode, but only 1 to 2 years after a lifting.

Minimal invasive apparented technology: radiofrequency ultrasound, cryolipolysis also create a tensing effect. Focalised ultrasounds (discontinuous type such as Ultra-shape®, or continuous type like Sonosculpt®, and recently Ulthera®), Shock Wave® using acoustic waves, endolasers using maily modes 1,604 and 980 nm, are being used in the facial region. It is often necessary to repeat the sessions. Their result is however still quite limited in these zones [36-39] Fig. 3.

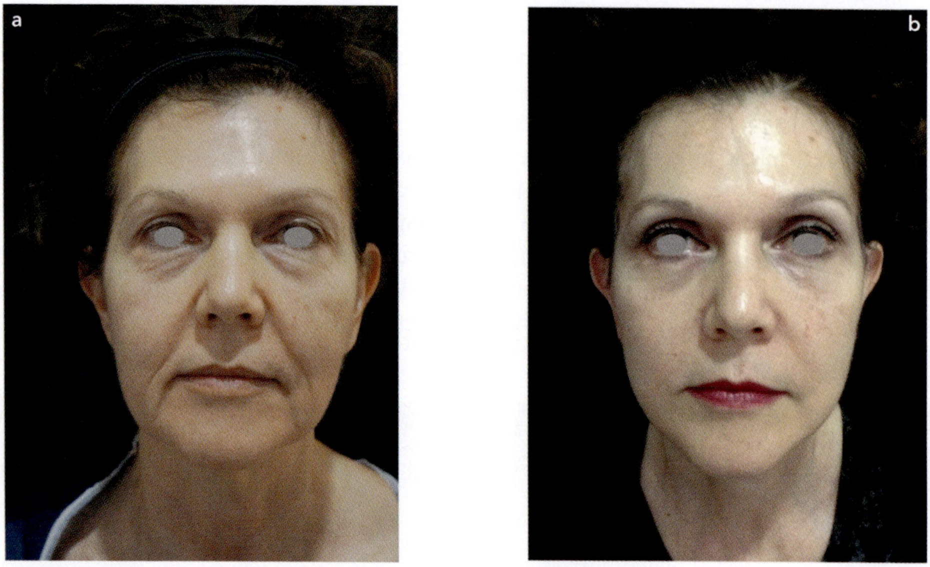

Figure 3 Cervico-facial lifting and blepharoplasty of 4 eyelids by CO_2 laser
(a) Before operation, result after 6 years (b)

Neck

Injection of the platysma bands is indicated either when the neck starts to age before the skin has become lax, or after a facelift which has not provided an effective solution on the front of the neck. If a decision has been made not to treat or re-treat the neck surgically, the toxin is a good indication [40-42].

When the depressor anguli oris muscle is particularly tonic and cause the corners of mouth to be pulled down, and when the permanent contraction of the platysma causes "ropes", a preventive treatment 3 weeks previous surgery seems to visibly improve the after-effects and results of the peribucal, oval as well as the neck areas. Study groups such as the one of Santini and Kestemont in Nice, France, have published promising preliminary results for platysma injections 3 weeks before a neck lift [3].

Laser and neck surgery: we already know the dangerous nature, as well as the side-effects of resurfacing lasers without surgery, especially in an ablative mode on the neck area. Resurfacing in this area should be performed with very specific constants that are adapted to the neck skin and in patients with a carefully selected profile, who will accept an often important erythematous reaction.

During neck lifting, ablative resurfacing laser should not be performed in a detached zone. Resurfacing which is made in the peribuccal area or the chin should be continued in the sub-mental zone in order to produce a harmonious transition.

Minimal invasive technologies: RF, ultrasound, cryolipolysis seem to have a more important effect on the neck zone than on the oval or mid-face level.

CONCLUSION

The combination of botulinum toxin with surgical treatments of the eyelids, facelifts of the upper and mid-third of the face, and surface medical treatments improves short- and long-term results.

In zones where lifting is not active, such as peribuccal and peripalpebral zones, laser and associated techniques effectively treat surface wrinkles and heliodermia spots (age spots, vascular legions, dilated pores, etc). In the same goal the prior injection of toxin before laser and injection of fillers optimize the results of these treatments [44-50].

The current trend is to use facelifts and blepharoplasties that are as minimally invasive as possible, and which provide remarkably effective and natural appearing results, combined with powerful but very safe medical techniques when used appropriately, such as botulinum toxin.

REFERENCES

[1] Goldman A. Combining procedures with botulinum toxin in plastic surgery. In: Hexsel D, Trindade de Almeida A, eds. Cosmetic use of botulinum toxin. Porto Alegre, Brazil: AGE Editora, 2002: 216-220.

[2] Fagien S. Intraoperative injection of botulinum toxin A into orbicularis oculi muscle for the treatment of crow's feet. Plast Reconstr Surg 2000; 105: 2226-2228.

[3] Ascher B, Landau M, Rossi B. Injection treatments in cosmetic surgery. Informa Healthcare, London. Editor 2008.

[4] Naoum C, Dasiou-Plakida D. Dermal filler materials and botulinum toxin. Int J Dermatol 2001; 40: 609-621.

[5] Coleman Moriaty K. Other solutions. Combination treatments. In: Coleman Moriaty K, ed. Botulinum toxin in Facial Rejuvenation. St Louis: Mosby, 2004: 128-129.

[6] Sommer B, Sattler G. Cosmetic indications according to anatomic region. In: Sommer B, Sattler G, eds. Botulinum toxin in Aesthetic Medicine. Berlin: Blackwell Science, 2001: Ch 3.

[7] Ascher B, Wibault-Collange C. Botulinum toxin (Dysport®) and hyaluronic acid (Hylaform®) association in the treatment of lines. A preliminary evaluation. Inamed Aesthet News 2002: n° 1.

[8] Ascher B. Toxine botulique et rides: les associations médicales et chirurgicales. Real Ther Derm Venerol 2004; 138: 7-9.

[9] Carruthers J, Carruthers A. A prospective, randomized, parallel group study analyzing the effect of BTX-A (Botox) and nonanimal sourced hyaluronic acid (NASHA, Restylane) incombination compared with NASHA (Restylane) alone in severe glabellar rhytides in adult female subjects: treatment of severe glabellar rhytides with a hyaluronic acid derivative compared with the derivative and BTX-A. Dermatol Surg 2003; 29: 802-809.

[10] Carruthers JDA, Carruthers A, Maberley D. Deep resting glabellar rhytides respond to BTX-A and Hylan B. Dermatol Surg 2003; 29: 539-544.
[11] Farks JP, *et al.* Effect of common laser treatments on hyaluronic acid fillers in a porcine model; Aesthetic Surg J 2008; 28: 503-511.
[12] Alam M, Levy R, Pavjani U, *et al.*; Safety of radiofrequency treatment over human skin previously injected with medium-term injectable soft-tissue augmentation materials: a controlled pilot trial. Lasers Surg Med 2006; 38: 205-210.
[13] Goldman, *et al.* A randomized trial to determine the influence of laser therapy, monopolar radiofrequency treatment, and intense pulsed light therapy administered immediately after hyaluronic acid gel implantation. Dermatol Surg 2007; 33: 535-542.
[14] Semchyshyn N, Kilmer S. Effect of non ablative rejuvenation laser treatment immediately following botox injection. Dermatol Surg 2005; 31 (S3): 399-404.
[15] West TB, Alster TS. Effect of botulinum toxin type A on movement-associated rhytides following CO_2 resurfacing. Dermatol Surg 1999; 25: 259-261.
[16] Yamauchi PS, Lask GP, Lowe NJ. Botulinum toxin type A gives adjunctive benefit to periorbital laser resurfacing. J Cosmet Laser Ther 2004; 6: 145-148.
[17] Nicolau PJ, Chaouat M, Mimoun M. Skin. Wrinkles and botulinum toxin. Ann Readapt Med Phys 2003; 46: 361-374.
[18] Borodic GE, Gozzolino D. Pharmacology and histology of therapeutic application of botulinum toxin. New York Marcel Dekker, 1994.
[19] Matsudo PK. Uso da toxina botulinica em estetica clinica e cirrurgica. Rio de Janero: Revinter, 2000: 279-281.
[20] Ascher B. Rajeunissement facial par lifting sans endoscopie et injection de toxine botulique. Objectif Peau 2000; 8: 158-161.
[21] Ascher B. Rides fronto-palpébrales: intérêt des injections de toxine botulique, du lifting sans endoscopie, du resurfacing laser. Cah Ophtalmol 1997; 14: 37-44.
[22] Ascher B, Rzany BJ, Grover R. Efficacy and safety of botulinum toxin type A in the treatment of lateral crow's feet: double-blind, placebo controlled, dose-ranging study. Dermatol Surg 2009; 35: 1478-1486.
[23] Ascher B, Zakine B, Kestemont P, *et al.* Botulinum toxin A in the treatment of glabellar lines: scheduling the next injection. Aesthet Surg J 2005; 25: 365-375.
[24] Ascher B, Zakine B, Kestemont P, Baspeyras M, Bougara A, Santini J. A multicenter, randomized, doubleblind, placebo-controlled study of efficacy and safety of 3 doses of botulinum toxin A in the treatment of glabellar lines. J Am Acad Dermatol 2004; 51: 223-233.
[25] Rzany B, Ascher B, Monheit G. Treatment of glabellar lines with botulinum toxin type A (Speywood unit) – A clinical overview. JEADV 2010; 24 (Suppl. 1): 1-14.
[26] Ascher B, Talarico S, Cassuto D, *et al.* International consensus recommendations on the aesthetic usage of botulinum toxin type A (Speywood Unit) – part I: upper facial wrinkles. JEADV 2010; 24 (11): 1278-1284.
[27] Ascher B, Talarico S, Cassuto D, Escobar S, Hexsel D, Jaén P, *et al.* International consensus recommendations on the aesthetic usage of botulinum toxin type A (Speywood Unit) – part II: wrinkles on the middle and lower face, neck and chest. JEADV 2010; 24 (11): 1285-1295.
[28] Guerrissi JO. Intraoperative injection of botulinum toxin A into orbicularis oculi muscle for the treatment of crow's feet. Plast Reconstr Surg 2000; 105: 2219-25 Plast Reconstr Surg 2003; 112 (Suppl): 161S-163S.
[29] Fagien S. Intraoperative injection of botulinum toxin A into orbicularis oculi muscle for the treatment of crow's feet. Plast Reconstr Surg 2000; 105: 2226-2228.
[30] Ahn MS, Catten M, Maas CS. Temporal brow lift using botulinum toxin A. Plast Reconstr Surg 2000; 105: 1129-35; discussion 1136-9.
[31] Huang W, Rogachefski AS, Foster JA. Browlift with botulinum toxin. Dermatol Surg 2000; 26: 55-60.
[32] Ahn MS, Catten M, Maas CS. Temporal brow lift using botulinum toxin A. Plast Reconstr Surg 2003; 112 (Suppl): 98S-104S.

[33] Maas C. Temporal brow lift using botulinum toxin A: an update. Plast Reconstr Surg 2003; 112 (Suppl): 109S-112S.
[34] Ortiz AE, Tremaine AM, Zachary CB. Long-Term Efficacy of a Fractional Resurfacing Device. Lasers Surg Med 2010; 42: 168-170.
[35] Ascher B, Landau M, Rossi B. Injection treatments in cosmetic surgery. Informa Healthcare, London. Editor 2008.
[36] Dahan S, Rousseaux I, Cartier H. Multisource radiofrequency for fractional skin resurfacing-significant reduction of wrinkles. J Cosm Laser Ther 2013; 15(2): 91-97.
[37] Laubach HJ, *et al.* Intense focused ultrasound: evaluation of a new treatment modality for precise microcoagulation within the skin. Dermatol Surg 2008; 34(5): 727-734.
[38] Weiss M. Commentary: noninvasive skin tightening: ultrasound and other technologies: where are we? Dermatol Surg 2012; 38 (1): 28-30.
[39] Alam M, *et al.* Ultrasound tightening of facial and neck skin: a rater-blinded prospective cohort study. J Am Acad Dermatol 2010; 62 (2): 262-269.
[40] Brandt FS, Bellman B. Botulinum A exotoxin for platysmal bands and rejuvenation of the aging neck. Dermatol Surg 1998; 24: 1232-1234.
[41] Matarasso A, Matarasso SL, Brandt FS, Bellman B. Botulinum A exotoxin for the management of the platysma bands. Plast Reconstr Surg 1999; 103: 645-652.
[42] Kane MA. Nonsurgical treatment of platysma bands with injection of botulinum toxin A. Plast Reconstr Surg 1999; 103: 656-663.
[43] Santini J, Kestemont P, Krastinova Lolov D. Chirurgie plastique de la face, rajeunissement, embellissement. Report of the Congrès de la Société Française d'Oto-Rhino-Laryngologie.
[44] Carruthers A, Cohen JL, Cox SE, De Boulle K, Fagien S, Finn CJ, *et al.* Facial aesthetics: achieving the natural, relaxed look. J Cosmet Laser Ther 2007; 9 [Suppl 1] 6-10.
[45] Semchyshyn NL, Kilmer SL. Does laser inactivate botulinum toxin? Dermatol Surg 2005; 31 (4): 399-404.
[46] Khoury JG, Saluja R, Goldman MP. The effect of botulinum toxin type A on full-face intense pulsed light treatment: a randomized, double-blind, split-face study. Dermatol Surg 2008; 34 (8): 1062-1069.
[47] Carruthers J, Carruthers A. The effect of full-face broadband light treatments alone and in combination with bilateral crow's feet botulinum toxin type A chemodenervation. Dermatol Surg 2004; 30 (3): 355-366.
[48] Landau M. Combination of chemical peelings with botulinum toxin injections and dermal fillers. J Cosmet Dermatol 2006; 5 (2): 121-126.
[49] Flynn TC, Carruthers J, Carruthers A. Botulinum-A toxin treatment of the lower eyelid improves infraorbital rhytides and widens the eye. Dermatol Surg 2001; 27 (8): 703-708.
[50] Carruthers J, Carruthers A. Aesthetic botulinum A toxin in the mid and lower face and neck. Dermatol Surg 2003; 29 (5): 468-476.

CHAPTER 13

Interactions between lasers, related technologies and injectable products

Bertrand Pusel

INTRODUCTION

According to the 2012 statistics from the ASAPS (American Society for Aesthetic Plastic Surgery), non-surgical aesthetic procedures have been evolving for around ten years and injections of botulinum toxin and fillers, the majority of which are based on hyaluronic acid, are two of the most commonly used techniques to treat the face.

In parallel, lasers are being widely used to manage facial skin aging, with a range of non-ablative and ablative technologies available, as are technologies that are considered related to lasers, such as radiofrequency and ultrasound.

Today facial rejuvenation is really only conceptualised in terms of combined techniques that bring together a number of treatment modalities. When lasers and other related treatments are used, irrespective of the technique chosen (ablative CO_2 laser, Erbium laser, ablative or non-ablative fractional lasers, RF, etc.), there are some anatomical areas that will see little or no improvement, such as the nasolabial folds, marionette lines, and the lip outline. Thus, these areas are treated by dermal fillers.

Similarly, the results of laser treatment will wear off over time in areas where the muscles are used for expression such as forehead wrinkles or crows' feet, indications that are best suited for treatment with botulinum toxin. It is appropriate to consider whether these different techniques have potential interactions, and whether it may be necessary to follow a specific treatment schedule.

HYPOTHESIS OF THE INTERACTION OF COMBINED TECHNIQUES

Lasers and other related techniques used to treat facial skin aging give rise to a two-pronged question concerning the depth at which they act and the temperature at which a thermal injury is produced. With regard to depth, tissue vaporisation using conventional ablative lasers for laser resurfacing generally reaches the superficial to mid-dermis.

With the advent of ablative or non-ablative fractional lasers, structures located deeper than one millimetre (i.e. the deep dermis) can be reached, while injected products are targeted directly. In terms of temperature, we know that many procedures induce a thermal injury that causes breakage of intermolecular cross-links of collagen at 63° C, which is the essential first step in the process of neocollagen generation, which is required for the treatment to be effective. This therefore introduces the problem of the thermo-lability of any other techniques used in combination.

We will build on the data found in literature regarding the use of botulinum toxin and dermal fillers in combination with treatments using lasers and other related technologies to treat the face.

INTERACTION WITH BOTULINUM TOXIN

Since this product is by definition injected into the muscle, it would logically seem to be "out of reach" of treatments using lasers and other related technologies.

The earliest studies of the interaction between laser treatments and botulinum toxin injections date from the time when laser resurfacing of the face using conventional ablative CO_2 or erbium lasers was being developed. Not only was an absence of negative interaction demonstrated, on the contrary, when the two techniques were used in combination, they produced a synergistic effect irrespective of the scheduling of the two procedures.

Yamaguchi [1] studied 33 subjects who underwent treatment of the periorbital area first with an injection of botulinum toxin and six weeks later with laser resurfacing. It was shown that this efficacy was superior on the side treated with both techniques. West [2] reached the same conclusions for a procedure in which botulinum toxin injections were carried out after laser resurfacing. In summary, when botulinum toxin is used in combination with laser resurfacing treatments, it leads to improved healing in the treated anatomical areas of expression lines, because the action of the toxin forces the muscles to rest. Similarly, the efficacy of the laser in the medium to long term is increased by regular botulinum toxin injections given around every six months, as is recommended in the good practice guidelines for use of this product.

In our experience, using these two techniques in combination produces remarkable results with optimal efficacy for the treatment of crows' feet, and to a lesser extent for the treatment of deep radial upper lip wrinkles, or "bar code lines".

In 2005, in a study on 20 subjects who underwent treatment to the glabella and crows' feet, Semchyshyn [3] reported that the efficacy of botulinum toxin injections at day 15 was not influenced by other treatments (pulsed dye laser, intense pulsed light, 1,540 nm laser remodelling, and radiofrequency) if the other treatment was administered only 10 minutes after the botulinum toxin injection.

Based on these results, we could conclude that there is a total absence of interaction with botulinum toxin even when it is performed virtually simultaneously with laser treatments or related technologies.

One should note that the fractional lasers have been developed since 2004 based on the concept of selective photothermolysis, and have not been assessed in the abovementioned studies. It has now been clearly established that significant oedema can follow treatments performed using non-ablative fractional lasers, especially in areas of thin skin such as the periorbital region. Thus, it has been suggested that there may be a risk of botulinum toxin migration with swelling, however this hypothesis has not yet resulted in a publication. Nonetheless, caution warrants allowing a two-week interval between procedures carried out using this kind of equipment and administration of a botulinum toxin injection.

INTERACTION WITH DERMAL FILLERS

Injectable dermal fillers made from hyaluronic acid (HA) have become the most commonly used products worldwide for the correction of static facial wrinkles.

There is a range of injection depths, and numerous injection techniques are described due to the sheer number of products available on the market: superficial treatments are based on the principles of mesotherapy or mesolift; treatments targeting the mid- or deep dermis aim to fill the main static facial wrinkles, and those reaching the subcutaneous tissue or even the bone structures, address facial volumizing. Other absorbable fillers such as calcium hydroxyapatite and poly-L-lactic acid are also in current use, and should be administered as a deep injection to produce a biostimulating effect.

In terms of clinical studies on humans, Goldman [4] considered 36 patients who were treated with two procedures. One was an injection of hyaluronic acid into the two naso-labial folds, and the other treatment was applied on one side only and randomly chosen from: intense pulsed light, 1,450 nm diode laser, 1,320 nmNd:YAG laser, or monopolar radiofrequency. The results of a blind evaluation showed that there was no difference in correction of the nasolabial folds between the two sides of the face (with or without laser treatment) at each point of follow-up (day 14, 28 and 56). Alam [5] performed a similar study using radiofrequency on the inner surface of the forearm and also concluded that there was no interaction.

However, as stated previously, the latest laser technologies, consisting of ablative or non-ablative fractional lasers have not been evaluated. In an attempt to answer this question, Farkas [6] used a porcine model to assess the influence of various systems after hyaluronic acid injection. No histological effect was demonstrated for the Sciton 560 nmIPL lamp, 1,064 nmNd:Yag laser, Lux 1,540 nm laser, or Active FX laser.

It was however noted that fractional ablative lasers (the Profractional™ fractional Erbium 2940 laser and DeepFX™ CO_2 laser) could interact immediately with dermal fillers injected superficially into the dermis with evidence of HA migration into the vaporisation micro-channels that have been created. The filler was however not noted to undergo any structural change.

Addressing related technologies, England [7] used a porcine model to evaluate the influence of radiofrequency after injection of several types of dermal fillers: hyaluronic acid, calcium hydroxyapatite, and poly-L-lactic acid. It was concluded that there was no change in the products at four months, and Shumaker [8] came to the same conclusion based on an experimental model.

The in vivo effect of lasers in general, and fractional lasers in particular on dermal filling products remains poorly documented. The thermal shock that laser or radiofrequency treatments induce does not seem to have any effect on dermal fillers, but doubts do persist on the long term maintenance of their performance since the majority of the studies published have considered results in the short or medium term only.

Further studies should be carried out in the near future to lift this uncertainty, making use of new techniques, such as sonography, to carry out the assessment. Sonography is able to determine the location of the filler and its depth in the skin. It can also be used for the opposite purpose to confirm whether a non-absorbable filling product has disappeared after laser treatment [9].

Denying that lasers have any influence would contradict the clinical observations recently reported by Cho [10], who demonstrated the efficacy of a 1,064 nm Q-switched laser to treat a Tyndall effect in a nasolabial fold after hyaluronic acid injection. This publication confirmed the results obtained by Hirsch [11], who had demonstrated a structural change to hyaluronic acid gel in a Petri dish during the period immediately following laser use.

Although the Tyndall effect may mean that the injection was too superficial, the fact remains that laser technology seems to be effective in modifying the structure of hyaluronic acid causing the lesion to disappear; nonetheless the mechanism of action for this effect of laser is still poorly elucidated, especially given that no chromophore can be easily evidenced in hyaluronic acid.

In summary, there is no consensus on the strategy to be adhered to when a laser treatment session is planned before or after injection of a dermal filler. Logic seems to suggest that, as far as possible when scheduling a patient's care, injections of dermal fillers should take place after any procedure using lasers or techniques that are considered related.

CONCLUSION

There is not enough data in literature to allow us to state that there is a complete absence of interaction between lasers and injectable treatments when these procedures are combined for the management of facial skin aging. Continuous interviews have led us to consider that the optimal treatment schedule starts with botulinum toxin injections, followed by treatment using lasers or other technologies that delivers energy, and ends with dermal fillers, with a suitable interval between the different procedures, especially in the case of ablative fractional lasers.

REFERENCES

[1] Yamaguchi PS, Lask GP, Lowe NJ. Botulinum toxin type A gives adjunctive benefit to periorbital laser resurfacing. J Cosmet Laser Ther 2004; 6: 145-148.
[2] West TB, Alster TS. Effect of botulinum toxin type A on movement-associated rhytides following CO_2 resurfacing. Dermatol Surg 1999; 25: 259-261.
[3] Semchyshyn N, Kilmer S. Effects of non ablative Rejuvenation laser treatment immediately following botox injection. Dermatol Surg 2005; 31-S3: 399-404.
[4] Goldman, *et al.* A randomized trial to determine the influence of laser therapy, monopolar radiofrequency treatment, and intense pulsed light therapy administered immediately after hyaluronic acid gel implantation. Dermatol Surg 2007; 33: 535-542.
[5] Alam M, Levy R, Pavjani U, *et al.* Safety of radiofrequency treatment over human skin previously injected with medium-term injectable soft-tissue augmentation materials: a controlled pilot trial. Lasers Surg Med 2006; 38: 205-210.
[6] Farkas JP, *et al.* Effects of common laser treatments on hyaluronic acid fillers in a porcine model. Aesthetic Surg J 2008; 28: 503-511.
[7] England LJ, Tan MH, Shumaker PR, *et al.* Effects of monopolar radiofrequency treatment over soft-tissue fillers in an animal model. Lasers Surg Med 2005; 37: 356-365.
[8] Shumaker PR, England JL, Dover JS, *et al.* Effect of monopolar radiofrequency treatment over soft tissue fillers in an animal model: part 2. Laser Surg Med 2006; 38(3): 211-217.
[9] Naouri M, Mazer JM. Résorption d'une accumulation de silicone après traitement par laser Fraxel non ablatif, objectivée par échographie cutanée haute résolution. Ann Dermatol Venerol 2013; 140(6-7): S205-S206.
[10] Cho SB, Lee SJ, Kang JM, Kim YY, Kiu DJ, Lee JH. Effective treatment of a injected hyaluronic acid-inducedtyndall effect with a 1,064 nm Q-switched Nd:YAG laser. Clin Exp Dermatol 2009; 34: 637-638.
[11] Hirsch RJ, Narurkar V, Carruthers J. Management of injected hyaluronic acid induced Tyndall effect. Laser Surg Med 2006; 38: 202-204.

CHAPTER 14

Cutaneous aging and cosmetology

Annick Pons-Guiraud

Over the past twenty years, considerable progress has been made in our understanding of the patho-physiological and molecular mechanisms of aging. This has led to the development of increasingly effective anti-aging products and has offered hope of other advances in the prevention and repair of the clinical signs of skin aging.

CUTANEOUS AGING

This is a very complex multifactorial process that combines:

– chronological aging, which is intrinsic, inevitable, and genetically determined although aggravated by free radicals and hormonal phenomena;

– extrinsic aging, an actinic process that is related to the harmful impact of cumulative exposure to ultraviolet and infrared light, which generates oxidative stress and is interconnected with environmental aging (tobacco, pollution, drugs, etc.) [1].

The epidermis shows thinning of the Malpighian layer, a process of accelerated keratinisation, increased desquamation following a disordered pattern, a thickened stratum corneum, and drying of the skin.

In the dermo-epidermal junction (DEJ) synthesis of collagen IV and VII decreases with age, as does tissue firmness. Although it starts out with an undulating shape, the DEJ gradually loses its curved appearance, stretching out and flattening, leading to lengthening of the skin.

In the dermis various dysfunctions trigger structural and functional changes. In intrinsic aging, the number, size and contractile activity of fibroblasts decreases, leading to reduced synthesis of extracellular matrix with deterioration of collagen and elastin fibres. The skin is thinner, drier, dehydrated, and discoloured [2].

The dermal changes seen in *photoinduced aging* (80% of cutaneous aging) are extremely accentuated. Oxidative stress, generated by repeated exposure to the sun's radiation, damages fibroblasts and activates matrix metalloproteinases.

Melanocytes are distributed in an irregular pattern along the basal membrane, which is why the complexion becomes uneven. The clinical signs of solar elastosis become visible: skin, that is at first thickened, later becomes very thin, all components of the integumentary system are dull, dry and rough, both discoloured spots and wrinkles multiply, especially around the lips, becoming gradually deeper, with vascular naevi and erythrosis completing this picture [3].

THE COSMETOLOGY OF AGING

It is essential to follow a few fundamental rules that are often neglected but which are necessary to limit and prevent the effects of aging on the skin.

Use of hygiene products

Twice-daily applications should be gentle (especially on mature skin), and include facial cleansing using a product for the correct skin type and lifestyle (outdoor sports, swimming, heavy consumption of food or wine, tobacco use, pollution, etc.).

Keep the face well hydrated

If the skin is well hydrated, the balance between the processes of cellular renewal and desquamation is maintained and this ensures that the skin can perform its function as a barrier. This requires both water intake through ingredients that are Natural Moisturising Factors or NMF (urea, allantoin, amino acids, hyaluronic acid, collagen, glycosaminoglycans, etc.), and retention of water transported from the deeper layers of the skin through aquaporins in order to limit imperceptible water loss, which is achieved through the application of lipid substances (cholesterol, triglycerides, and especially ceramides) meaning that in this way the skin barrier is maintained.

Avoid or limit exposure to the sun

The harmful effects of the free radicals produced are well-known [4].

Lead a healthy lifestyle

Eat a sensible diet, exercise, stop or limit consumption of tobacco, alcohol, and drugs.

ACTIVE ANTI-AGING AGENTS

These are becoming increasingly numerous and are often combined within one cosmetic product; they mainly combat free radicals but they must also stimulate cellular synthesis (collagen/elastin).

Retinoids [5]

Topical retinoic acid (vitamin A acid) causes effects like irritation, erythema, desquamation, and a burning sensation. For these reasons, its precursors are preferred [6].

Retinol improves fine lines caused by both natural aging and photoaging by stimulating keratinocyte proliferation and collagen, elastin and fibronection production, increasing glycosaminoglycan (GAG) levels and causing matrix metalloproteinase (MMP) levels to fall [7].

Retinaldehyde has been tested for efficacy on actinic aging through imprinting and surface profilometry [8]. A reduction in wrinkles is noted as well as a smoothing and firming effect, since it induces a significant rise in numbers of keratinocytes, stimulates involucrin and transglutaminase, and triggers epidermal hyperplasia that is associated with a significant increase in CD44 receptors for hyaluronic acid (HA), which is why the combination of retinaldehyde and HA is so useful in stopping and improving skin aging [9].

Alpha hydroxy acids

These molecules have hydrating properties at low concentrations, and are exfoliating agents at a slightly higher concentration (over 12%). They have effects on both the dermis and epidermis through increasing GAG and collagen and elastin synthesis. Because of this they reduce fine lines and sometimes wrinkles, returning radiance to dull and aged mature skin [10].

Hyaluronic acid (HA)

When incorporated in the form of small low MW fragments or combined with a saponin, HA reduces cutaneous atrophy by stimulating keratinocytes and protecting dermal collagen [11].

Vitamins

B3 or nicotinamide improves the signs of photoaging, reduces photo-induced elastosis by increasing the synthesis of sphingolipids, free fatty acids, cholesterol and ceramides thus strengthening the skin barrier. In addition, it inhibits the transfer of melanosomes to keratinocytes, reducing hyperpigmentation [12].

B9 or topical folic acid protects keratinocytes after exposure to UV radiation and boosts repair of UV damage to DNA.

Vitamin C (L-ascorbic acid) levels fall with age, especially in the epidermis. Controlled studies have confirmed that when it is applied topically, it improves the clinical appearance of photo-aged skin and reduces facial wrinkles. It is an anti-inflammatory and antioxidant, stimulating collagen production and acting on MMP. Furthermore, it causes depigmentation because it inhibits tyrosinase [13].

Vitamin E from the sebaceous glands is naturally present at the skin surface and it is the main soluble antioxidant in the membrane lipids. Once it has been oxidised, vitamin

E can be regenerated in its reduced form by vitamin C, which is why there are numerous formulations that combine vitamins C and E in order to boost the skin's endogenous antioxidant defences against the free radicals generated by exposure to UV rays.

There are also other ingredients with anti-free radical properties:

Sirtuins, so-called "longevity" proteins, repair damage to DNA and RNA and are stimulated by some compounds such as resveratrol; phytohormones (soya isoflavones), some enzymes (glutathione peroxidase, catalase, superoxide dismutase), trace elements (Zn, Se, Mn), and carotenoids (carotene, lycopene) stimulate tissue regeneration; algae provide amino acids, vitamins, mineral salts, and trace elements; anti-glycant agents (silicon and derivatives) fight the stiffening actions of collagen and elastin. Numerous plant extracts are increasingly incorporated into cosmetics, and contain active anti-aging ingredients including centella asiatica, which encourages tissue regeneration.

The efficacy of anti-wrinkle products is evaluated using a variety of clinical and instrumental, qualitative or quantitative methods [14]:

– the qualitative/clinical methods involve a direct intra-individual comparison using in vivo subjects or later using standardised photographs. These methods are reasonably reliable;

– quantitative/instrumental methods quantify the effects of anti-wrinkle products in terms of the change in cutaneous relief with regard to microdepressions, which are measured by the depth of the furrows. They are performed either by direct contact, making moulds or imprints that are then analysed, usually by optic profilometry, or without contact, in vivo, through fringe projection followed by image processing.

Sensory analysis applied to anti-aging products

Sensory measures connected to the olfactory, gustatory, visual, tactile, or temperature receptors take a hedonic and analytical approach and they are used as a guide in the formulation of cosmetic products. The consumer's overall perception of a product is based on the unconscious analysis of the collection of stimuli received by the somesthetic or kinaesthetic sensory receptors [15].

Organic cosmetics

Organic cosmetics are highly esteemed by the public because the ingredients used in the formulations are safe. In France, these products must meet "the three specifications" that are additional to the official regulations governing cosmetics and are defined by the organisations Ecocert, Qualité France, Nature and Progrès. They guarantee that all plant ingredients used are grown organically (no chemical fertiliser, pesticides, insecticides, or synthetic herbicides) and that there is a high natural ingredient content (95%), as well as the absence of parabens, silicon, PEG and GMO, respect for the environment throughout the whole production chain, and precise percentages stated on cartons and packaging.

Chemical peels

Although these methods have been around for many years, chemical peels are useful in the overall management of cutaneous aging. The range of peels is diverse and highly developed, and they are indicated in the aging of facial skin as a whole, wrinkles and fine lines, patches of discolouration, and actinic keratosis. Depending on the exfoliant and the concentration, peels can be:

- light or very light: TCA 10-35%, AHA 35-70%, SA 50%;
- medium: TCA 35-50% possibly combined with Jessner's solution.

These treatments can induce neocollagen production that leads to a smoothing and rejuvenating effect;

- deep: Phenol 50, 55%, which is a peel that sometimes has a difficult recovery period and a trained operator is required. This technique may be limited to use on the area around the mouth Fig. 1.

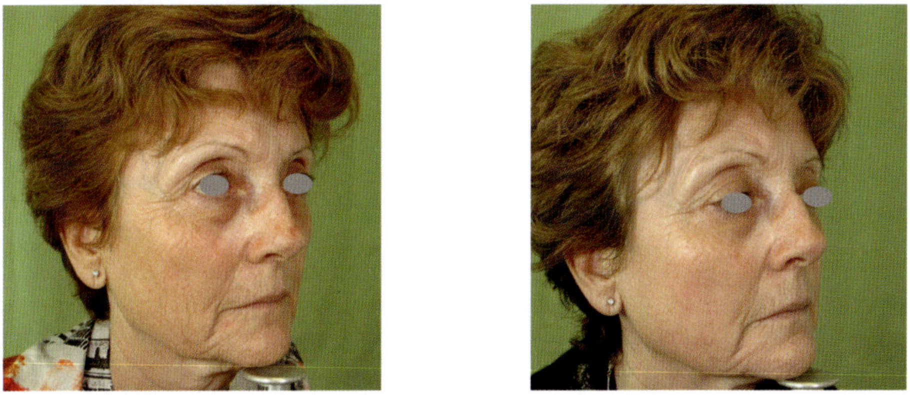

Figure 1 Improvement in chronological aging with a 30% trichloroacetic acid peel *(photos M. Baspeyras)*

IN ADDITION TO A TOPICAL SKINCARE ROUTINE

Lasers

In view of the diversity of lasers available, they are very useful for the correction of skin aging. Ablative lasers (CO_2, Erbium) remain a very effective treatment for significant photoaging but this invasive technique is increasingly being replaced by non-ablative lasers (Fraxel) Fig. 2.

Although less effective, collagen-remodelling lasers are also useful and are non-invasive.

There are techniques other than lasers, such as intense pulsed light, LED, and radiofrequency, which also have their place in the correction of skin aging.

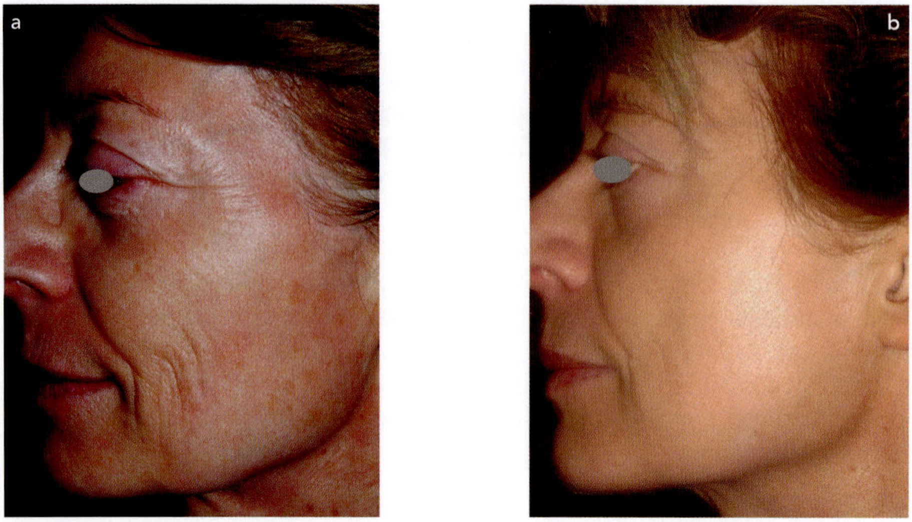

Figure 2 Improvement in actinic aging with non-ablative fractional laser (Fraxel) treatment
Before treatment (a), result after 4 months (b).
(photos J.-M. Mazer)

Mechanical stimulation

This approach is particularly useful because over the course of the aging process fibroblasts lose contractility and mechanical function, which encourages a reduction in collagen synthesis and organisation, leading to skin slackening. The positive effect of this mechanical stimulation on the fibroblasts is evidenced by the increase in synthesis of cytokines, growth factors, and extracellular matrix proteins as well as the increased length of the DEJ and thickness of the epidermis, which is completed by improved viscoelasticity and more radiant skin [16, 17].

Chronobiology of anti-aging products

The skin is subject to a 24-hour circadian rhythm. The epidermis must provide daytime protection against external assaults (UV, pollution, stress), while regenerating and repairing itself during the night. This is why a day cream is necessary, to be applied before 1 pm, and why a night cream applied at bedtime is effective, given that maximum mitosis takes place in the epidermis at 1 am and the absorption peak of these substances occurs at 4 am.

Pharmaceutical preparation of the product

This is a determining factor for efficacy, safety and acceptability and these depend on a number of parameters:

– the availability and stability of active ingredients, as well as whether they are compatible and complementary;

– the vehicle chosen to transport the active ingredients to their target;

– the formulation being suitable for the skin type: water in oil for dry skins, oil in water for oily skins;

– the form of the presentation: emulsion, microemulsion, multilamellar vesicles, encapsulated forms, silicon-based forms, oils, and very recently nanoemulsions and hydrogels which are widely used to encourage hydration and improve stratum corneum quality.

Cosmetovigilance

Clear cosmetovigilance must be ensured. Any mild or serious side effect due to a cosmetic product must be declared, in France, to ANSM (French National Agency for the Safety of Medicines and Health Products) and as far as possible, the ingredient responsible must be identified and labelled.

WHICH AREAS WILL BE STUDIED AND DEVELOPED IN THE COSMETOLOGY OF TOMORROW?

Stem cells are the pillars of cutaneous regeneration. These undifferentiated cells with the capacity for unlimited self-renewal account for fewer than 1% of cells in the stratum basale, but they decline with age leading to slower renewal of the epidermis [18]. However, they are surrounded by a specialised and protected microenvironment that preserves their undifferentiated qualities and their integrity. In cosmetology, there are also attempts to maintain their vitality and capacity for division by acting on protecting their microenvironment but rather than using stem cells of human origin, whose behaviour it is not yet prudent to modify, active cosmetic ingredients of plant origin are preferred, extracted using biotechnologies. Some of these known as "plant stem cells" have exceptional powers of self-regeneration as well as providing the necessary elements to protect cutaneous stem cells (examples are the leaves of rock samphire, wild pear, buddleja, etc.).

– The reconstruction or stabilisation of telomeres and the study of progerin to ensure DNA protection are developments that are particularly anticipated [19].

– The study of the structure, metabolism, and biological role of glycans is another fundamental subject in the study of aging because when glycan levels fall with age this leads to cells becoming locked, blocking the processes that maintain youth.

– Developing models of reconstructed, ex vivo, or even in vitro skin would allow for an even better study of the characteristics of aging skin and the effects of the different oxidative stressors, including environmental factors, and from there the prevention or slowing of the skin aging process.

– Other subjects for study: the neutralisation of the phenomenon of glycation, new innovations in formulations, and improvements in the presentation of cosmetic products.

CONCLUSION

Dr Faustus's fantasy is getting closer to becoming a reality...

REFERENCES

[1] Beylot C. Vieillissement cutané: aspects cliniques, histologiques et physiopathologiques. Annales de dermatologie 2009; 136, supplément 6: S263-S269.
[2] Okano Y, Masaki H, Sakurai H. Dysfunction of dermal fibroblasts induced by advanced glycation endproducts (AGEs) and the contribution of a non-specific interaction with cell membrane and AGEs. J Dermatol Sci 2002; 29: 171-180.
[3] Stoebner PE, Meunier L. Photo-vieillissement du visage. Ann Dermatol Venereol 2008; 135: 1S21-6.
[4] Sauvaigo S, Bonnet-Duquennoy M, Odin F, *et al.* DNA repair capacities of cutaneous fibroblasts: effects of the sun exposure, age and smoking on response to an acute oxidative stress. Br J Dermatol 2007; 157: 26-32.
[5] Sorg O, Antille C, Kaya G, Saurat JH. Retinoids in cosmeceuticals. Dermatol Ther. 2006; 19: 289-96.
[6] Darlenski R, Surber C, Fluhr JW. Topical retinoids in the management of photodamaged. Skin: from theory to evidence-based practical approach. Br J Dermatol 2010; 163: 1157-1165.
[7] Kang S, Duell EA, Fisher GJ, *et al.* Application of retinol to human skin in vivo induces epidermal hyperplasia and cellular retinoid binding proteins characteristic of retinoic acid but without measurable retinoic acid levels or irriation. J Invest Dermatol 1995; 105: 549-556.
[8] Saurat JH, Didierjean L, *et al.* Topical retinaldehyde on human skin: biologic effects and tolerance. 1994; 103: 770-774.
[9] Cordero A, Leon-Dorantes G, Pons-Guiraud A, *et al.* Retinaldehyde/hyaluronic acid fragments: a synergistic association for the management of skin aging. J Cosmet Dermatol 2011; 10: 110-117.
[10] Gougerot-Schwartz A. Alpha-hydroxyacides et vieillissement cutané. Encycl Méd Chir. Cosmétologie et Dermatologie Esthétique 2000; 50-160-12: 7 p.
[11] Kaya G, Tran C, Sorg O, Hortz R, *et al.* Hyaluronate fragments reverse skin atrophy by a CD44-dependent mechanism. PloS Med 2006; 3(12): e493.
[12] Bissett DL, Oblong JE, Berge CA. Niacinamide: AB vitamin that improves aging facial skin appearance. Dermatol Surg 2005; 31: 860-865.
[13] Humbert PG, Haftek M, Creidi P, *et al.* Topical ascorbic acid on photoaged skin. Clinical, topographical and ultrastructural evaluation: double-blind study vs. placebo. Experimental Dermatology 2003; 12: 237-244.
[14] Turlier V. Evaluation de l'efficacité des produits antirides. Keratin 2012; 18: 14-19.
[15] Rolin G, Placet V, Jacquet E, Humbert P. Development and characterization of a human dermal equivalent with physiological mechanical properties. Skin Res Technol 2012 May; 18(2): 251-258.
[16] Varani J, Dame MK, Rittie L, *et al.* Decreased collagen production in chronologically aged skin: roles of age-dependent alteration in fibroblast function and defective mechanical stimulation. Am J Pathol 2006; 168: 1861-1868.
[17] Won-Serk Kim, Byung-Soon Park, Jong-Hyuk Sung. Protective role of adipose-derived stem cells and their soluble factors in photoaging. Arch Dermatol Res 2009; 301: 329-336.
[18] Prat M, Leclerc T, Thépenier C, *et al.* Intérêt des cellules stromales mésenchymateuses dans le traitement des brulures cutanées. Stem Cell Res Ther 2012 May 31; 3(3): 20.
[19] Cao K, Blair CD, Faddah DA, *et al.* Progerin and telomere dysfunction collaborate to trigger cellular senescence in normal human fibroblasts. J Clin Invest 2011; 121: 2833-2844.

CHAPTER 15

The objective evaluation of the effects of laser treatment in skin aging

Michael Naouri

Lasers and related techniques are widely used in the management of skin aging. The current trend relies on less invasive techniques but the counter-argument claims that the results are more difficult to see, and often develop gradually over time. These constraints mean that new tools needed to be developed that attempt to objectively show the true effect of these treatments, in order to comply with the principle of evidence-based assessment. Faced with a lack of specific instruments, the dermatologist has to be creative and borrow skin imaging and engineering technologies from the cosmetics industry (biometrology). These techniques are valuable because they offer the possibility to obtain objective results in vivo and without trauma. These results are at once sensitive, specific, and they can quantify the effects of treatment. These assessment methods are also useful for carrying out comparative studies on the different treatment modalities, and for meeting patients' requirements for objective monitoring of their treatment. The choice of technique will depend on local availability, finances, and the purpose of the assessment: improvement of colour or texture, dermal changes, treating laxity.

THE INSTRUMENTS IN THE DERMATOLOGY CLINIC "TOOLBOX"

This toolbox consists of all the techniques that are normally used in the practice of dermatology, and does not need any specific investment to be made.

Digital photography is the most commonly used assessment tool. The advantage of using a camera is that it is readily available, the examination is quick to carry out, and an immediate comparison can be made. There are numerous software packages available for processing digital photos. Their value in optimising comparisons during the consultation is clear: cropping, optimising brightness, colour, etc. Filters can also be useful to assess any changes in colour. However, the use of these editing tools is not permitted for most science journals in order to ensure objectivity through the absence of "retouched" images. One possible alternative is to use photos with colorimetric scales or a colour test chart, which may allow for a better assessment of vascular and pigmented lesions. There will be numerous constraints on obtaining good quality images: reproducing positioning or exposure, or the need to use the same camera for all of the shots because the results from different cameras can vary. Ultimately, it is often necessary to invest in a mini photographic laboratory when good quality images are desired. The other drawback of digital photography is that by definition it renders a three-dimensional shape into two dimensions, so it is difficult to show the efficacy of techniques such as skin tightening.

There are other techniques used in dermatology that could be useful for assessing laser treatments although they do have limitations in that they are subjective and do not offer quantifiable results: *dermatoscopy* can be used to analyse the impacts of laser treatments, certain areas of microrelief (such as size of dilated pores) and pigmentation, while a *Wood's lamp* can show dermal and epidermal pigmentation, and *polarised light* can visualise vessels Fig. 1.

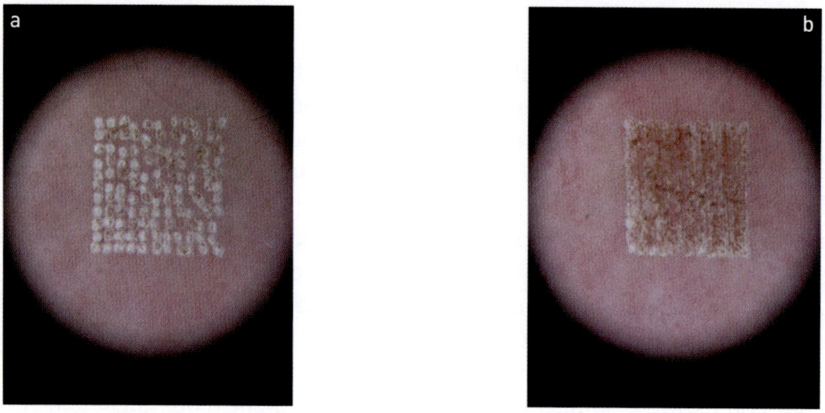

Figure 1 Use of dermatoscopy to demonstrate the distribution of the microimpacts of fractional CO_2 laser: an even spacing with random distribution (a) will keep the effect of overlapping thermal injury to a minimum (b)

HISTOLOGY TO EVALUATE LASER TREATMENTS

A skin biopsy is the logical extension of numerous interventions in dermatology. Its use in assessing anti-aging techniques can only be discussed in the context of clinical studies. This is of course an invasive procedure that routinely risks development of a permanent scar. The standard histological exam will offer information about the immediate effect of the laser on the skin: visualisation of the ablated area and the peripheral thermal damage in fractional laser treatment, immediate effect on pigments and vessels, etc. As part of the treatment monitoring, a pathology assessment can follow the changes induced until the final result is achieved, which is usually synthesis of neocollagen and reorganisation of the extracellular matrix in procedures to manage skin aging, followed by pigment extrusion or changes in vascularisation after treatment.

Immunohistochemistry techniques can be used to complete the examination, consisting of using antibodies targeted against specific proteins whose presence will demonstrate the stimulation that occurs after laser treatment [1, 2]: heat shock proteins (HSP), collagen type 1 or 3, procollagens, elastin, vascular endothelial growth factors, etc. Other techniques, such as electron microscopy to examine the ultrastructure, can show reorganisation of the fibres of the dermal extracellular matrix. The main limitations of histological examination are that it correlates poorly with clinical features: neocollagen synthesis or an increase in heat shock proteins do not necessarily translate into improved skin quality, and even less so into a reduction in wrinkles; only small surface areas can be assessed due to the size of the punch biopsy; the data obtained is qualitative rather than quantitative.

BIOMETROLOGY TO ASSESS LASER TREATMENTS

Use of these techniques will often require a substantial investment so they are really only suitable for dermatology practices or centres, which are willing to become involved in clinical trials.

Measuring colour

There are two main elements that determine skin colour: the skin's vascularisation and its pigmentation. Colour can be converted into objective coordinates that can be defined using the L*a*b colour space system, as set out by the International Commission on Illumination. This system is made up of two perpendicular horizontal axes using complementary colours: a (red-green) and b (yellow-blue); and a vertical axis representing lightness: L (white-black). Absolute measurements can be taken using a spectrocolorimeter or spectrophotometer, while relative measurements are taken with the tristimulus method (*Chromameter*®). Relative spectrophotometry can be used to look only at the wavelengths that are useful for studying the skin (*Mexameter*® and *DermaSpectrophotometer*®). Colorimetric measurements are particularly valuable for monitoring the vascular or pigment changes caused by aging [3, 4] as well as for assessing the safety of treatments by measuring the erythema triggered, or assessing reactive pigmentation [5].

Measuring elasticity

Analysing the biomechanical properties of the skin is a relatively complex process because its structure consists of three layers of different thicknesses, which are composed of elements with multiple biomechanical properties (the epidermis consists of the lamellar structure of the *stratum corneum* and mucous bodies of the Malpighian layer; the dermis contains collagen, elastin, glycosaminoglycans and fibroblasts; the subcutis is made up of adipocytes and fibrous septae, etc.). The measurements obtained are very often relative and they depend on the measuring instrument. The *Cutometer®* Fig. 2 has managed to establish itself in the medical literature as being the gold standard tool [6]. This instrument studies the outcome of a suction-induced skin deformation, and a time-deformation curve is produced.

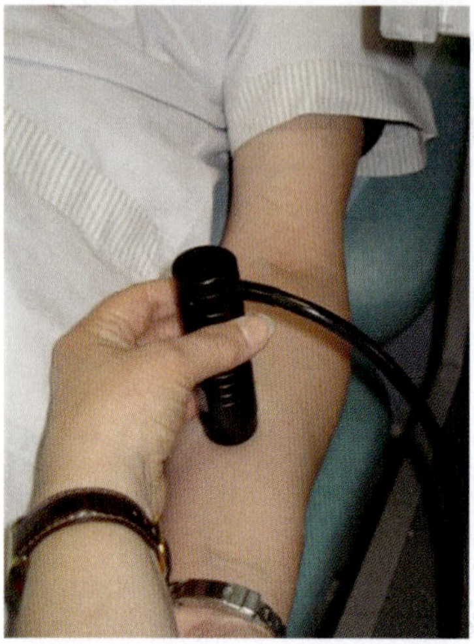

Figure 2 Using a cutometer

Today, a computerised assessment has supplanted the formal study of this curve, and this process leads to more reliable parameters that represent the main biomechanical properties of the skin: elasticity in the true sense, meaning the capacity to respond to stretching by returning to the original position, which mainly depends on dermal elastic and collagen fibres; viscoelasticity, meaning the tendency to retain the deformation like modelling clay ("loss of firmness"), which is primarily related to the hydration capacity brought about by glycosaminoglycans; and fatigability after repeated cycles of suction. These cutaneous fatigability parameters can be correlated with a decrease in the tendency of the skin to produce expression lines. Other instruments are also available that use ultrasound beams (*Echorheometer®*) or that study the effect of torsion (*Dermal Torque Meter®*).

It is particularly useful to analyse elasticity parameters in order to evaluate the systems for treating skin tightening. We have recently shown that the effect of lasers on elasticity parameters is variable over time. This means that while elasticity initially seems to be improved after treatment with fractional CO_2 laser [7], an objective follow-up of changes on cutometry shows subsequent dermal stiffening that can be demonstrated through a paradoxical loss of elasticity [8].

Measuring relief

Numerous techniques are available for assessing the relief of the skin. The standard methods that have been widely used by the cosmetics industry make use of replicas (*mechanical or optical profilometry*) or in vivo analysis through *beam projection*. Recent usage of three-dimensional film is undeniably a step forward in terms of cost and ease of use, and this type of measurement could ultimately be popularised through encouraging its accessibility to dermatologists. An analysis of relief is useful when evaluating photorejuvenation techniques [5, 9] by looking at the reduction in wrinkles and lines and the superficial microrelief (pores and other structural abnormalities).

Other measurements

There are other biometrology approaches that can be useful for the assessment of laser techniques [5]. The Sebumeter® has been used to show the reduction in sebum after laser remodelling. Similarly, tools to measure hydration (*Corneometer®*, *Evaporimeter®*, *Tewameter®*, etc.) can be useful to study the safety of treatments. A pH meter could be an objective assessment of treatments for sweating.

SKIN IMAGING

High-resolution ultrasonography of the skin Fig. 3

High-resolution ultrasonography of the skin is probably one of the most useful tools for the objective monitoring of laser treatments for aging. Unlike other sonography systems, these machines analyse what is happening in the skin rather than passing through the skin. This is made possible by a ceramic transducer, which means the exploration can use of high frequencies (between 16 and 25 MHz). This high-resolution obtains remarkably accurate measurements, correlated to histology [11]. Sonography of the skin can make a close analysis of global dermal changes in thickness and density and any solar elastosis in the SENEB (Sub Epidermal Non Echogenic Band). Several studies have shown the dermis to increase in thickness and density after treatment with fractional lasers or laser remodelling, with no changes in the SENEB [8, 9, 11]. Since sonography of the skin produces accurate quantifiable results, it is useful in setting up a statistical analysis as it produces criteria by which the response to laser treatment can be determined [8, 11]. It has also been possible to show that young and thin skins respond better to fractional CO_2 laser, and that the effect of treatment was not governed by prior application of anaesthetic EMLA cream, or the regularity of follow-up after the intervention [11]. Another use for sonography of the skin is the objective and quantitative monitoring of dermal changes over time, which has shown progressive improvement in skin quality after treatment up to the sixth month [8]. Finally, if a dermal filler injection has been used first, sonography can identify the location of the filler and its depth in the skin with the purpose of attempting to keep laser-filler interactions to a minimum. The technique can also be used for the opposite purpose, to confirm whether a non-absorbable filling product has disappeared after laser treatment [12].

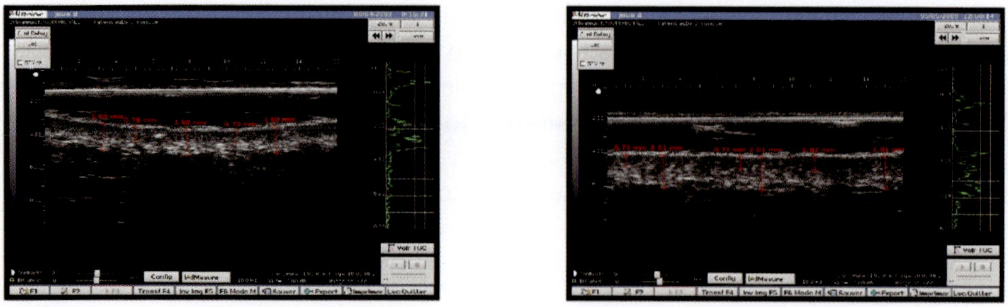

Figure 3 High-resolution sonography of the skin: dermal thickening after fractional CO_2 laser

Other imaging techniques

Other skin imaging techniques such as optical coherence tomography and confocal microscopy have also been used in the assessment of skin aging. Although these tools have significant resolution, they cannot be used to explore structures located deeper than the papillary dermis [13]. Confocal microscopy can be used to study the dermoepidermal junction, measured by the index of dermal papillae (number of papillae per mm^2), which tends to fall with age. This index may be improved after fractional laser treatment [14].

CONCLUSION

Assessment tools mean that subjectivity is eliminated in the evaluation of laser treatments for aging, and they are indispensable in terms of granting studies scientific credibility. Nonetheless, since these techniques are extremely sensitive, this could risk a paradoxical focus on measurements that are statistically significant but clinically irrelevant. This means that these tools must be correlated with clinical assessment in order to keep any risk of bias to a minimum.

REFERENCES

[1] Hantash BM, Bedi VP, Kapadia B, Rahman Z, Jiang K, Tanner H, Chan KF, Zachary CB. In vivo histological evaluation of a novel ablative fractional resurfacing device. Lasers Surg Med 2007 Feb; 39(2): 96-107.
[2] Laubach HJ, Tannous Z, Anderson RR, Manstein D. Skin responses to fractional photothermolysis. Lasers Surg Med 2006 Feb; 38(2): 142-149.
[3] Li YH, Wu Y, Chen JZ, Gao XH, Liu M, Shu CM, Dong GH, Chen HD. Application of a new intense pulsed light device in the treatment of photoaging skin in Asian patients. Dermatol Surg 2008 Nov; 34(11): 1459-1464.
[4] Koh BK, Lee CK, Chae K. Photorejuvenation with Submillisecond Neodymium-Doped Yttrium Aluminum Garnet (1,064 nm) Laser: A 24-Week Follow-Up. Dermatol Surg 2010 Mar; 36(3): 355-362.
[5] Christian MM. Microresurfacing using the variable-pulse erbium:YAG laser: a comparison of the 0.5- and 4-ms pulse durations. Dermatol Surg 2003 Jun; 29(6): 605-611.

[6] Dobrev H. Study of human skin mechanical properties by mean of cutometer. Folia Med (Plovdiv) 2002; 44: 1-5.
[7] Naouri M, Atlan M, Perrodeau E, Georgesco G, Khallouf R, Martin L, Machet L. Skin tightening induced by fractional CO_2 laser treatment: quantified assessment of variations in mechanical properties of the skin. J Cosmet Dermatol 2012; 11(3): 201-206.
[8] Naouri M, Perrodeau E, Martin L, Machet L. Laser CO_2 fractionné: suivi objectif, sur une période de six mois, des modifications dermiques induites par échographie cutanée haute résolution et cutométrie (Évaluation Objective des Lasers en Esthétique [EOLE] 3). Ann Dermatol Venerol 2012; 139(12): B76.
[9] Fournier N, Dahan S, Barneon G, Rouvrais C, Diridollou S, Lagarde JM, Mordon S. Nonablative remodeling: a 14-month clinical ultrasound imaging and profilometric evaluation of a 1,540 nm Er:Glass laser. Dermatol Surg 2002; 28: 926-931.
[10] Machet L, Belot V, Naouri M, Boka M, Mourtada Y, Perrinaud A, Giraudeau B. Preoperative mesurement of thickness of cutaneous melanoma using high-resolution 20 MHz ultrasound imaging: feasibility and peatfalls to predict surgical margins, a prospective study of 31 cases and a systematic review. Ultrasound Med Biol 2009; 35(9): 1411-1420.
[11] Naouri M, Atlan M, Perrodeau E, Georgesco G, Khallouf R, Martin L, Machet L. High-resolution ultrasound imaging to demonstrate and predict efficacy of carbon dioxide fractional resurfacing laser treatment. Dermatol Surg 2011; 37(5): 596-603.
[12] Naouri M, Mazer JM. Résorption d'une accumulation de silicone après traitement par laser Fraxel® non ablatif, objectivée par échographie cutanée haute résolution. Ann Dermatol Venerol 2013; 140(6-7): S205-S206.
[13] Sattler EC, Poloczek K, Kästle R, Welzel J. Confocal laser scanning microscopy and optical coherence tomography for the evaluation of the kinetics and quantification of wound healing after fractional laser therapy. J Am Acad Dermatol 2013; 18.
[14] Shin MK, Kim MJ, Baek JH, Yoo MA, Koh JS, Lee SJ, Lee MH. Analysis of the temporal change in biophysical parameters after fractional laser treatments using reflectance confocal microscopy. Skin Res Technol 2013; 19(1): e515-e520.

CHAPTER 16

Particularities of facial rejuvenation with laser and related technologies in Asian skin

Nark-Kyoung Rho

INTRODUCTION

When treating skin of different types using laser and other energy-based devices, we have to understand that there are fundamental differences in skin histology, in patterns of aging and in risk factors for skin aging, and the nature of the complications.

BIOLOGY AND HISTOLOGY OF THE ASIAN SKIN

A hallmark biologic feature in people with skin of color is the amount and epidermal distribution of the cutaneous pigment, melanin [1]. It is well established that irrespective of skin color, humans all have the same number of melanocytes. However, at the level of the ultrastructure of the skin, the melanosomes in lighter skin are smaller and aggregated in complexes whereas in darker skin, there are larger melanosomes. The melanosomes of the Caucasians are grouped or aggregated together within a surrounding membrane. The melanosomes of the East Asian subjects are likewise grouped in aggregates but the configuration is more compact, compared with those of the Caucasoid subjects. Asian skin exposed to sunlight has a predominance of non aggregated melanosomes, whereas unexposed skin has predominately aggregated melanosomes [1]. Skin color differs greatly even among Asian subjects. According to the study by Galzote *et al.* [2], which compared the skin properties of 100 female subjects each from a total of eight Asian cities in China, India, Korea, Japan, and the Philippines, skin color was darkest in the subjects from Calicut (southern India) and fairest in those from Sendai (northern Japan) demonstrating a direct relationship between the melanin content and the average amount of the sun exposure received by the skin.

There is conflicting data regarding racial differences in stratum corneum structure. There are some studies suggesting that the stratum corneum in darker skin is more compact than in fair skin. Other epidermal structures are not much different in Asians and Caucasians. There are evidences suggesting no significant differences in sweat glands between races. Racial differences in sebaceous gland size and activity have been suggested [1]. The hair of Asian subjects, as demonstrated in Chinese people, is the closest in shape to a circular section, and with the largest cross-sectional area. In contrast, the hair of Western European subjects was found to have the smallest cross-sectional area [3]. Under electron microscopy, the size of isolated melanin granules from the hair of black subjects was found to be larger than those from the hair of fair-skinned and Asian (Chinese) subjects [1]. Despite these differences, the hair of members from all races share common structural elements.

Dermal fibroblasts in dark-skinned female facial skin are larger and occurrs in greater quantity compared with those in white female facial skin. The actual collagen fiber bundles in dark-skinned individuals are smaller, more closely stacked, and run more parallel to the epidermis. In addition, many collagen fibrils and glycoprotein fragments are noted in the dermal interstices and throughout the dermis [1]. This may partly explain the higher incidence of keloid in Asian and black populations.

Maximum reflectivity of skins for three different wavelengths, i.e. 694, 775, and1,064 nm is higher in Caucasians than Asians [4]. Generally speaking, Asian skin is less prone to laser light reflection and scattering than Caucasian skin because the relative abundance of chromophores in Asian skin absorbs a larger fraction of the irradiated laser light. Thus, the photon density in the skin is less influenced by other laser-tissue interactions Fig. 1. The abundance of skin chromophores, especially melanin, causes problems when treating cutaneous vascular lesions using short-wavelength laser or light systems (e.g., long-pulse 532 nm lasers, intense pulsed light systems with short cut-off filters) so caution is required when treating telangiectasia or port-wine stains in darkly pigmented Asian patients using these systems.

SKIN BARRIER FUNCTION IN ASIAN PATIENTS

Kompaore *et al.* [5] showed that trans-epidermal water loss (TEWL) measurements were higher in Asians and Blacks compared to Caucasians. Tape stripping increased TEWL more in Asians compared to Caucasians. After repetitive stripping, the order of skin sensitivity was: Asian > Caucasian > black, which means that the removal of the stratum corneum increases skin permeability, with racial differences. After sodium lauryl sulfate testing, Aramaki *et al.* [6] found significant subjective sensory differences between Japanese and German women, i.e., Japanese women complained about stronger irritation. This may imply a faster penetration of irritants in Asian females. An increased

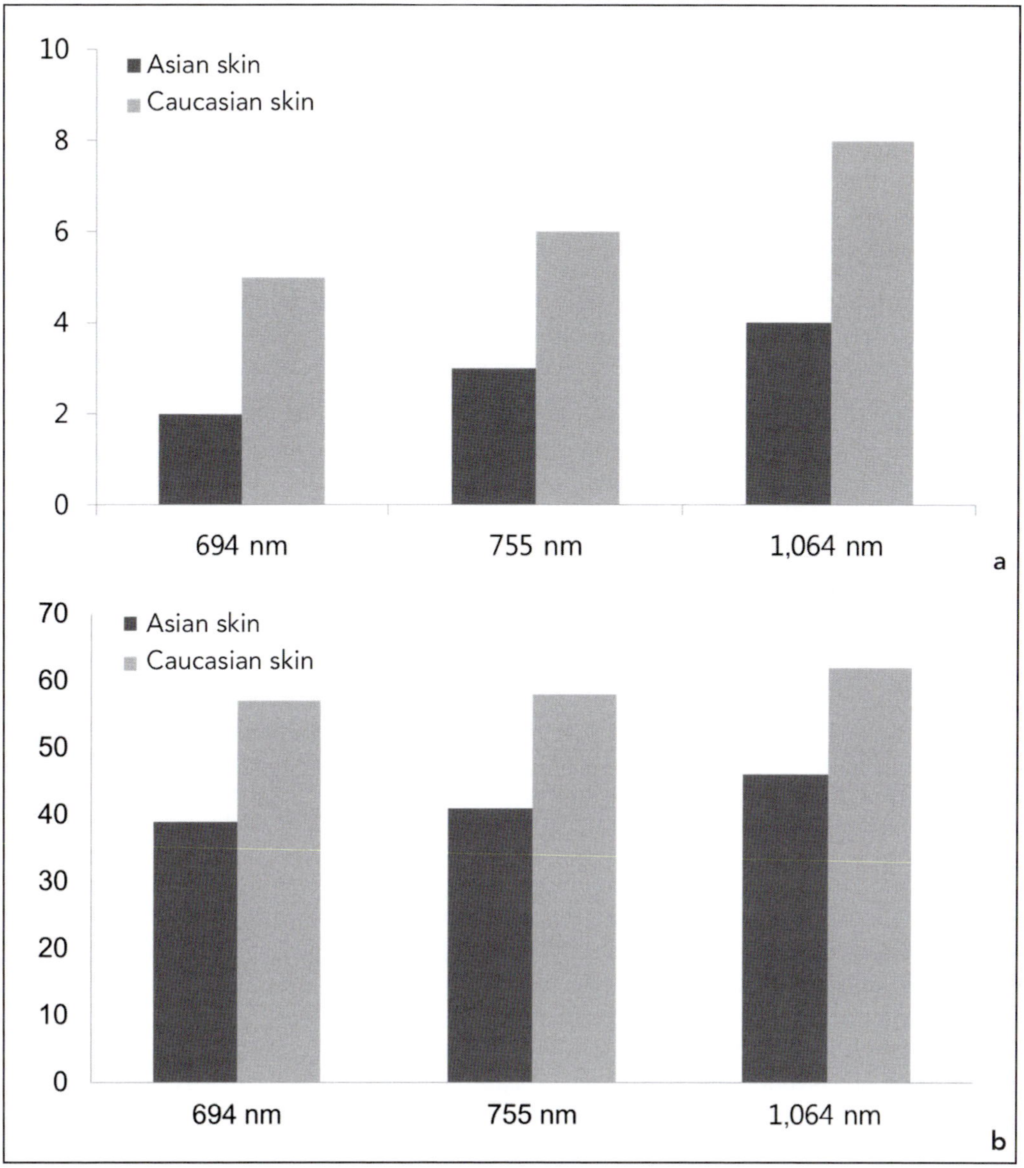

Figure 1 Maximum scattered beam width (a) and maximum reflectivity of backscattered light (b) in Asian skin and Caucasian skin according to the wavelength (modified from [4])

reactivity was noted for Asian versus Caucasian subjects for irritants in another comparative study [7]. In fact, the incidence of irritation to cosmetics, standard positive irritants, capcaisin, and retinol appeared significantly higher in Asian than in Caucasian subjects [8]. It is generally believed that Asian skin is more sensitive than Caucasian skin. However, small sample sizes, external variability and intra-variability within the subgroups in studies make it difficult to firmly conclude this. Given that virtually all energy-based facial treatments are related to a temporary increase of TEWL, it is mandatory to give appropriate skin hydration after procedure in Asians. In fact, active moisturization after laser treatment (either ablative or non ablative) is a standard regimen in many East Asian countries.

PAIN THRESHOLD

Rahim-Williams *et al.* [9] conducted a systematic literature review of 472 studies using experimental pain stimuli to assess pain sensitivity across multiple ethnic groups and concluded that Asians show similar or slightly lower pain threshold than non-Hispanic Caucasians whereas African Americans tended to demonstrate the lowest pain tolerance. Usually female patients experience more pain than male patients.

AGING OF THE ASIAN SKIN

One of the hallmarks of photoaging in East Asians is pigmentation. It has been reported that the patterns of pigmentary change that occur in Asians are dependent on gender [10]. Lentigo increases with age, and is more frequent in women than in men. On the other hand, seborrheic keratosis also increases with age, and this is more common in men [10, 11]. As a benign tumor, seborrheic keratosis is not a pigmentary disorder. However, because most seborrheic keratosis lesions in Asians are pigmented, both patients and physicians in Asia regard seborrheic keratosis as a pigmentation problem [12]. Seborrheic keratoses are observed in 80-100% of people over 50 years in Korea [12]. One study [13] demonstrated that cumulative sunlight exposure is an independent contributory factor of the development of seborrheic keratosis in aging Asian males. Freckling (ephelides), which is most frequent in Caucasians with red or blond hair and blue eyes, appears to be less common in Asians [12]. Melasma is a common pigmentary disorder in all Asian races Fig. 2. There seems to be a tendency that Indian, Thai, and Malay subjects have more widespread types of melasma than Chinese, Korean, and Japanese people. Unlike reports based on the Caucasian patients, fractional laser resurfacing does not provide good results in Asian patients with melasma. Aggressive fractional laser treatment often causes aggravation of the condition.

Many people believe that wrinkles are not a prominent feature of photoaged Asian skins, and that dyspigmentation is a major manifestation in Asian skins. However, a statistically significant positive association between wrinkling and dyspigmentation has been found in both Asian women and men [12]. This suggests that Asians with severe dyspigmentation usually tend to have severe wrinkles; smoking, sun exposure, and female sex are independent risk factors for wrinkles in this subgroup. Natural defense mechanisms against sun exposure include the production of melanin, the thickening of the stratum corneum and the presence of epidermal proteins, such as urocanic acid [12]. Nevertheless, the development of wrinkles in Asians is not as early, fast, and severe as in Caucasians. In a study [14] that compared Chinese and French populations, there was a decade delay in the development of wrinkles in Chinese populations. Goh [15] reported that wrinkling in Asians is not noticeable until the age of about 50, and that even then

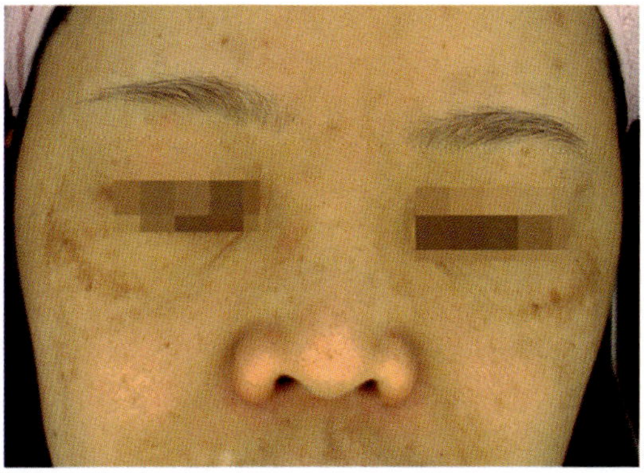

Figure 2 Melasma is a very common pigmentary disturbance in Asian women

its degree is not as marked as in Caucasian subjects of a similar age. In Asians, visible wrinkles usually do not present before 30 years of age and they become apparent from the age of 50 [12]. The wrinkle scores in the forehead, glabella, upper eyelid, and corner of the eye were similar at advanced ages between East Asian females and Caucasian females, while the wrinkle scores in lower eyelid, nasolabial folds, cheek, and corner of the mouth were markedly higher in Caucasian females than in Japanese females, and reached an upper limit at advanced ages in Caucasian females [16]. The sagging score was significantly higher in Caucasian females than in Japanese females in the groups aged 40 years or more. Delayed skin aging in Asian people might be related to the antioxidant defense enzyme levels in the skin. There are some data that show catalase activities of Asian subjects are higher than those of Caucasians [17].

Nevertheless, histologic signs of photoaging (e.g., epidermal atrophy, cell atypia with poor polarity, and disorderly keratinocyte differentiation) have been observed in the skin of Asian subjects as well. Deeply or darkly pigmented skin still experiences photodamage, as evidenced by pigmentation disorders and other signs of epidermal and dermal damage, although they "age better" than people with white skin [1]. The primary difference between Caucasian and Asian skin is attributed to melanocytic function. As Asian skin is more highly pigmented, its acute and chronic cutaneous responses to UV irradiation differ from those of white skin [12]. Chung *et al.* [10] found that wrinkling patterns in Asians differ from those of Caucasians. Asians have coarser, thicker and deeper wrinkles, particularly on the forehead, perioral and crow's feet areas. In contrast, Caucasians usually have relatively fine wrinkles on their cheeks and the crow's feet area. Within a race, some people develop severe skin wrinkling while others develop mild skin wrinkling, although they have the same risk factors. This observation suggests the possibility that there may be wrinkle-associated genes or single nucleotide polymorphisms (SNPs) in certain genes, such as collagen, elastin or matrix metalloproteinase (MMP) genes. Further investigations on photoaging-related genes are required to understand such racial and individual differences in terms of susceptibility to skin wrinkling. In general, Asian patients who have coarse wrinkles and prominent skin pores respond less to the conventional fractional laser rejuvenation, radiofrequency skin tightening, or high-intensity ultrasound skin lifting procedures compared to Caucasian elderly patients whose skin is thinner and wrinkles are fine.

It has been reported that in the brown skin of Thai, Malay, and Indian races, changes in pigmentation seem to be a more important feature in prematurely aged skin than wrinkling [12]. Skin wrinkling in these populations is not readily apparent until the age of about 50 years, and even then the degree of wrinkling is not as marked as in Caucasian skin [12]. In one intra-Asian comparative study [18], female subjects in Bangkok showed the most severe level of wrinkles, followed by those in Shanghai and in Tokyo. Interestingly, significant differences were observed between Thai and Japanese women in the intensity of wrinkles at many facial sites. Chinese women had significantly more wrinkles around the eyes compared to Japanese women, while Thai women had significantly more wrinkles in the lower halves of their faces compared to Chinese women. In a similar study [19], Singaporean (Chinese) women had the highest cheek skin elasticity compared to Indonesian and Vietnamese women and Vietnamese women's elasticity was the lowest. These results indicate variations in skin aging features among women from three Asian cities thereby suggesting the diversity of Asian skin.

CHANGES OF MELANOCYTES AND PIGMENTATION IN PHOTOAGED ASIAN SKIN PRONE TO HELIODERMY

The number of dopa-positive melanocytes in human skin decreases with age by approximately 10-20% with each decade in both habitually sun-exposed and protected skin [20]. Despite decreased melanocyte density with aging, photoaged skin shows irregular pigmentation and, frequently, hyperpigmentation. This may be due to a higher level of DOPA activity in chronically irradiated melanocytes [12]. Heterogeneity of skin color in exposed areas of elderly skin is due to an uneven distribution of pigment cells, a local loss of melanocytes, and modified interactions between melanocytes and keratinocytes [21].

In Korean brown skin, researchers [12] have found that the number of melanocytes in sun-exposed facial skin is greater than that of sun-protected buttock skin where the number of melanocytes decreases with aging. In photoaged facial skin, DOPA activity was greater and the number of melanocytes higher with aging. The amount of melanin pigment in the sun-exposed Asian skin was greater than that in sun-protected skin on an individual basis. Melanin pigment tended to decrease slightly in sun-protected buttock skin of Asians with aging, and localized mainly in the basal cell layer. On the other hand, in sun-exposed skin, the melanin pigment appeared to increase with aging, and to extend to the upper spinous layers beyond the basal cell layer. In this regard, daily use of sunscreens and other photoprotective methods are important for Asian skin mainly for the prevention of UV-induced pigmentary changes.

WHITENING COSMETICS PROBLEMS IN ASIA

In many parts of Asia, especially in south-eastern countries, there is a predilection for fair skin. This leads to some people using dangerous, illegal, compounded products with very high concentrations of hydroquinone or fluorinated steroids. A desire for soothing of lines and wrinkles is not as strong as the desire for "skin whitening" in this subcontinent. Sometimes, legally approved cosmetic whitening products cause serious problems, but this remains a rare occurrence. Recently one of the most famous Japanese cosmetics maker announced it was recalling 54 skin whitening products from all over Asia (Japan and 10 Asian territories: Taiwan, Hong Kong, South Korea, Thailand, Singapore, Malaysia, Indonesia, Myanmar, the Philippines and Vietnam) due to the fact that it was related with the development of leucoderma-like lesions [22] Fig. 3.

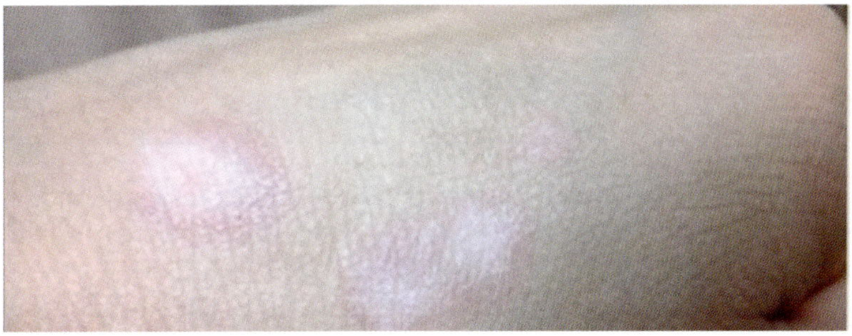

Figure 3 Whitening cosmetics-related side effects frequently cause dermatological and social problem in many Asian countries

FITZPATRICK SKIN TYPES

Fitzpatrick skin typing (Tab. 1) is still a controversial issue in Asia. For example, East Asians are typically labeled as having skin types III to V, but when looking at their response to sun we see a large variation. Many East Asian females tell dermatologists that they usually burn in sunlight but tan minimally. This would clearly make their skin classified as a type two, even though they may have relatively darker skin. The ethnicity of a patient is probably a better hallmark of classification than true Fitzpatrick types.

Table 1 Fitzpatrick skin types

Type	Description
I	Always burns, never tans (pale white skin)
II	Always burns easily, tans minimally (white skin)
III	Burns moderately, tans uniformly (light brown skin)
IV	Burns minimally, always tans well (moderate brown skin)
V	Rarely burns, tans profusely (dark brown skin)
VI	Never burns (deeply pigmented dark brown to black skin)

According to the study by Youn *et al.* [23], the most frequent skin type in Korea was type III (48.8%), followed by IV (22.2%) and V (17.8%). The skin type III was the predominant skin type in both men and women in Korea. However, skin type IV was found more frequently in men and there was a tendency that frequency of skin type IV and V increases with advancement of age. Interestingly, 11.2% of the study subjects were classified as having sun-sensitive skin types (types I and II).

Although every condition can occur in each ethnicity, post-inflammatory hyperpigmentation (PIH) is probably the most important issue in Asians whereas solar elastosis, actinic damage and rosacea, which are the most common problems in Caucasians, are less prevalent in Asians. In East Asia, dermatosis papulosanigra is not as prevalent as in Polynesia or Africa, although the exact incidence is not known. Pigmentation issues such as melasma are frequent in all Asian population. However, infraorbital darkening tends to be more common in Indian people than in East Asians.

POST-INFLAMMATORY HYPERPIGMENTATION

PIH is more common in darker skin types. For example, a fair-skinned patient acne tends to present post-acne erythema and atrophic scarring whereas in darker subjects, PIH and nodular scarring are more frequent sequelae of acne. PIH can also be caused by treatment, either medical or surgical. In Asians, it is not uncommon to notice a development of PIH even with the needle puncture during filler injections, not to mention the laser treatment Fig. 4.

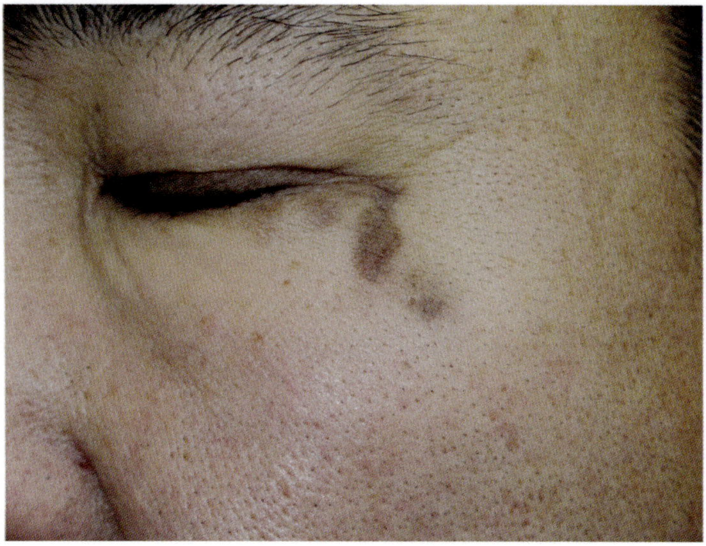

Figure 4 Post-inflammatory hyperpigmentation after 532 nm Q-switched Nd:YAG laser treatment of senile lentigo in a Korean male patient

The author [24] performed a retrospective clinical analysis on the development of post-Q-switched laser PIH in Korean female patients with freckles (n = 115) or senile lentigos (n = 175). The incidence of PIH after laser treatment was 34.1% and the most commonly involved area was forehead (63.5%) and temples (61.2%) followed by perioral (50.0%), preauricular (48.8%), malar (20.3%), and submalar (14.3%) areas. PIH developed more frequently in the senile lentigo group than in the freckle group (relative risk, RR = 2.77), during spring/summer season than during autumn/winter season (RR = 2.03), in older patients (> 45 years) than in younger patients (RR = 1.84), respectively. Pre-

and post-laser vitamin C iontophoresis showed a preventive effect on the development of PIH (RR = 0.49). Negishi *et al.* have [25] reported that aggressive irradiation using Q-switched 532 nm Nd:YAG lasers resulted in a high PIH incidence, while having no advantage in efficacy. For darker skin types, mild irradiation reduces the PIH risk with no disadvantage in efficacy. Wang *et al.* [26], have shown that the severity of laser PIH in Asian skin was lower in the 4-mm spot with a lower fluence than in the 3-mm spot with a higher fluence in patients with lentigines ($p = 0.03$) and concluded that using a larger spot to achieve the same biologic effect at a lower fluence is associated with equal efficacy and less severe PIH. Intense pulsed light (IPL) has been found to be related to significantly lower risk of PIH than Q-switched laser in the treatment of freckles and lentigines in Asian skin [27].

Various treatments have been used for the laser-induced PIH, although none of the existing therapies yields an entirely satisfactory outcome [24]. Standard therapies include monotherapy with topical retinoids, tretinoin in combination with hydroquinone and dexamethasone, and chemical peels. Chemical peels are regarded to work best when used in combination with topical bleaching regimens. Given the propensity of darker skin types to develop PIH, superficial peels are more suitable than medium-depth or deep chemical peels in terms of minimizing complications [28]. A recent randomized, controlled study [29] comparing the incidence of PIH between topical antibiotic and topical antibiotic with corticosteroid showed that application of topical steroid immediately after laser treatment has a tendency to halt hyperpigmentation and erythema without side effects. Newer treatment modalities for PIH in Asian patients include the use of 1,064 nm Q-switched Nd:YAG laser with low fluence and large spot size [30]. Although the precise mechanism of therapeutic effects of this treatment on PIH still remains to be elucidated, the concept of "subcellular selective photothermolysis" has been postulated [31]. Too aggressive or repetitive treatment can cause hypopigmentation Fig. 5.

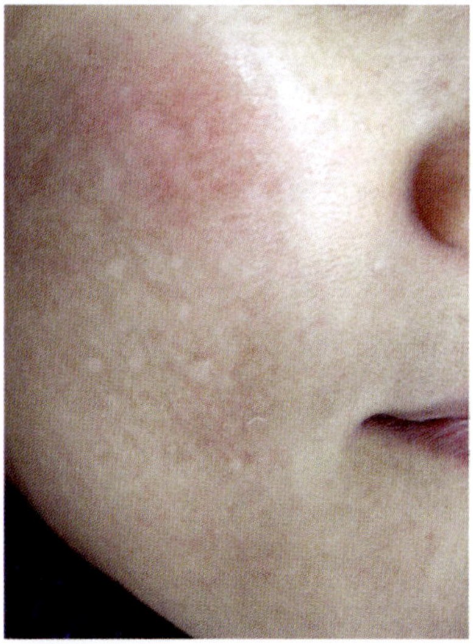

Figure 5 Mottled hypopigmentation after low-fluence 1,064 nm Q-switched Nd:YAG laser therapy for the treatment of melasma in a Korean female patient

SOUTH-EAST ASIAN SKIN

Although data on the skins of East Asians (Chinese, Korean, and Japanese) have been regularly presented, few studies have examined the skin of South-East Asians. Indeed, South-East Asians are composed of various ethnic backgrounds. For example, the population of the Philippines results from centuries of intermarriage between Chinese, Spanish and Malays so the Filipino skin is different from that of Malayan Indonesians or Malaysians [32]. Further studies are required to directly compare South-east Asian skin with East Asian skin, with emphasis on the response to the laser treatment.

CONCLUSION

Although basic biological and histological properties are not much different among different ethnic groups, the hallmarks of aging Asian skin differ from those of Caucasian's, and the relative risks of each aggravating factor may also differ. These clinical differences make primary and secondary response of their skin to laser and related technologies differ from that of Caucasian patients. More investigation is needed on the inherent characteristics of Asian skin, and on the aging and photoaging processes in Asians.

REFERENCES

[1] Taylor SC. Skin of color: biology, structure, function, and implications for dermatologic disease. J Am Aca Dermatol 2002; 46(2 Suppl Understanding): S41-S62.

[2] Galzote C, Estanislao R, Suero MO, Khaiat A, Mangubat MI, Moideen R, *et al.* Characterization of facial skin of various Asian populations through visual and non-invasive instrumental evaluations: influence of age and skincare habits. Skin research and technology: official journal of International Society for Bioengineering and the Skin 2013; 19(4): 454-465.

[3] Vernall DG. A study of the size and shape of cross sections of hair from four races of men. Am J Phy Anthropol 1961; 19: 345-350.

[4] Ansari M, Massudi R. Study of light propagation in Asian and Caucasian skins by means of the boundary element method. Optics Lasers Engin 2009; 47(9): 965-970.

[5] Kompaore F, Marty JP, Dupont C. In vivo evaluation of the stratum corneum barrier function in blacks, Caucasians and Asians with two noninvasive methods. Skin pharmacology: the official journal of the Skin Pharmacology Society 1993; 6(3): 200-207.

[6] Aramaki J, Kawana S, Effendy I, Happle R, Loffler H. Differences of skin irritation between Japanese and European women. British J Dermatol 2002; 146(6): 1052-1056.

[7] Robinson MK. Population differences in acute skin irritation responses. Race, sex, age, sensitive skin and repeat subject comparisons. Contact Dermatitis 2002; 46(2): 86-93.

[8] Lee E, Kim S, Lee J, Cho SA, Shin K. Ethnic differences in objective and subjective skin irritation response: an international study. Skin research and technology: official journal of International Society for Bioengineering and the Skin 2013.

[9] Rahim-Williams B, Riley JL, 3rd, Williams AK, Fillingim RB. A quantitative review of ethnic group differences in experimental pain response: do biology, psychology, and culture matter? Pain Med 2012; 13(4): 522-540.
[10] Chung JH. The effect of sunlight on the skin of Asians. Comprehensive Series in Photosciences 2001; 3: 69-90.
[11] Chung JH, Lee SH, Youn CS, Park BJ, Kim KH, Park KC, *et al.* Cutaneous photodamage in Koreans: influence of sex, sun exposure, smoking, and skin color. Arch Dermatol 2001; 137(8): 1043-1051.
[12] Chung JH. Photoaging in Asians. Photodermatology, photoimmunology & photomedicine 2003; 19(3): 109-121.
[13] Kwon OS, Hwang EJ, Bae JH, Park HE, Lee JC, Youn JI, *et al.* Seborrheic keratosis in the Korean males: causative role of sunlight. Photodermatology, photoimmunology & photomedicine 2003; 19(2): 73-80.
[14] Nouveau-Richard S, Yang Z, Mac-Mary S, Li L, Bastien P, Tardy I, *et al.* Skin aging: a comparison between Chinese and European populations. A pilot study. J Dermatol Sci 2005; 40(3): 187-193.
[15] Goh SH. The treatment of visible signs of senescence: the Asian experience. British J Dermatol 1990; 122 Suppl 35: 105-9.
[16] Tsukahara K, Fujimura T, Yoshida Y, Kitahara T, Hotta M, Moriwaki S, *et al.* Comparison of age-related changes in wrinkling and sagging of the skin in Caucasian females and in Japanese females. J Cosm Sci 2004; 55(4): 351-371.
[17] Yamashita Y, Okano Y, Ngo T, Buche P, Sirvent A, Girard F, *et al.* Differences in susceptibility to oxidative stress in the skin of Japanese and French subjects and physiological characteristics of their skin. Skin pharmacol physiol 2012; 25(2): 78-85.
[18] Tsukahara K, Sugata K, Osanai O, Ohuchi A, Miyauchi Y, Takizawa M, *et al.* Comparison of age-related changes in facial wrinkles and sagging in the skin of Japanese, Chinese and Thai women. J Dermatol Sci 2007; 47(1): 19-28.
[19] Lee MR, Nam GW, Jung YC, Park SY, Han JY, Cho JC, *et al.* Comparison of the skin biophysical parameters of Southeast Asia females: forehead-cheek and ethnic groups. J Europ Aca Dermatol Venereol: JEADV 2012.
[20] Quevedo WC, Szabo G, Virks J. Influence of age and UV on the populations of dopa-positive melanocytes in human skin. J Investig Dermatol 1969; 52(3): 287-290.
[21] Ortonne JP. Pigmentary changes of the aging skin. British J Dermatol 1990; 122 Suppl 35: 21-28.
[22] Japan's Kanebo recalls cosmetics over skin stain fears. AFP. 2013 July 3.
[23] Youn JI, Choe YB, Park SB, Suh DH, Park YK, Ahn SK, *et al.* The Fitzpatrick skin type in Korean people. Korean J Dermatol 2000; 38(7): 920-927.
[24] Rhee DY, Park GH, Rho NK, Chang SE. The prediction and prevention of laser-induced post-inflammatory hyperpigmentation. Korean J Cosmet Dermatol 2012; 9(1): 38-41.
[25] Negishi K, Akita H, Tanaka S, Yokoyama Y, Wakamatsu S, Matsunaga K. Comparative study of treatment efficacy and the incidence of post-inflammatory hyperpigmentation with different degrees of irradiation using two different quality-switched lasers for removing solar lentigines on Asian skin. J Europ Aca Dermatol Venereol: JEADV 2011.
[26] Wang CC, Chen CK. Effect of spot size and fluence on Q-switched alexandrite laser treatment for pigmentation in Asians: a randomized, double-blinded, split-face comparative trial. J Dermatol Treat 2012; 23(5): 333-338.
[27] Wang CC, Sue YM, Yang CH, Chen CK. A comparison of Q-switched alexandrite laser and intense pulsed light for the treatment of freckles and lentigines in Asian persons: a randomized, physician-blinded, split-face comparative trial. J Am Aca Dermatol 2006; 54(5): 804-810.
[28] Soriano T, Grimes PE. Postinflammatory Hyperpigmentation. Color Atlas of Chemical Peels: Springer; 2012. p. 143-8.
[29] Uaboonkul T, Nakakes A, Ayuthaya PK. A randomized control study of the prevention of hyperpigmentation post Q-switched Nd:YAG laser treatment of Hori nevus using topical fucidic acid plus betamethasone valerate cream versus fucidic acid cream. Journal of cosmetic and laser therapy: official publication of the European Society for Laser Dermatology 2012; 14(3): 145-149.

[30] Cho SB, Park SJ, Kim JS, Kim MJ, Bu TS. Treatment of post-inflammatory hyperpigmentation using 1064-nm Q-switched Nd:YAG laser with low fluence: report of three cases. J Europ Aca Dermatol Venereol: JEADV 2009; 23(10): 1206-1207.
[31] Kim JH, Kim H, Park HC, Kim IH. Subcellular selective photothermolysis of melanosomes in adult zebrafish skin following 1064-nm Q-switched Nd:YAG laser irradiation. J Investig Dermatol 2010; 130(9): 2333-2335.
[32] Jacinto S, Langle S, Noblesse E, Bonnet-Duquennoy M, Bernois A, Bonté F, *et al.* Architectural characteristics of sun exposed and sun protected south-east Asian skin. Int J Cosm Science 2005; 27(1): 44-46.

CHAPTER 17

Particularities of the management of dark skin

Ashraf Badawi

INTRODUCTION

People with dark skin, also referred to as skin of color or pigmented skin, constitute a wide range of racial and ethnic groups, including Africans, African Americans, African Caribbeans, Chinese and Japanese, Native American Navajo Indians, certain groups of fair-skinned persons (e.g., Indians, Pakistanis, Arabs), and Hispanics. It has been predicted that people with skin of color will constitute a majority of the United States and international populations in the 21st century.

The published literature supports a racial differential in epidermal melanin content and melanosome dispersion in people with dark skin compared with fair-skinned people. Other studies have demonstrated differences in hair structure and fibroblast size and structure between dark and fair-skinned people. These differences could at least in part account for the lower incidence of skin cancer in certain people of color compared with fair-skinned people; a lower incidence and different presentation of photo aging; pigmentation disorders in people with skin of color. However, biologic or genetic factors are not the only elements impacting on these differences in dermatology practice. Cultural practices can also have a significant impact [1].

DEFINING SKIN OF COLOR

The Skin Phototype (SPT) system has been used classically by dermatologists to categorize all people, including those with pigmented skin. This system, developed by Fitzpatrick, is predicated on the reactions or vulnerability of various types of skin to sunlight and ultraviolet radiation (UVR) [2,3]. It correlates the color of skin with its dynamic ability to respond to UV light with burning or tanning. This classification system was developed to categorize white skin; all skin of color was initially classified as skin type V. Obviously, skin of color encompasses greater color gradations. Subsequently, skin of color was divided into 3 groups: type IV, V, and VI. It is widely accepted in the dermatologic community that an individual with an olive skin tone, also characterized as beige or lightly tanned, is classified as having type IV skin, those with brown skin as type V, and black skin as type VI. These skin types rarely or never burn on sun exposure and tan readily. They include individuals of many racial and ethnic backgrounds. A majority of African Americans, Caribbean Americans, and Hispanic Americans would therefore be classified as having Fitzpatrick skin types IV through VI. Furthermore, there are many Asian Americans (e.g. Vietnamese and Koreans) and even fair-skinned persons (e.g. Arabs, Pakistanis, Indians) who also would be classified as having types IV and V skin.

The Lancer Ethnicity Scale (LES) is a classification system designed to calculate healing efficacy and durations in patients undergoing cosmetic laser or chemical peel procedures [4]. The patient's skin color is an important factor to consider in assessing the risk involved with such procedures.

Individuals with dark skin might be better served by a skin classification system based on criteria other than sensitivity to UV radiation or healing efficacy. For instance, a classification system based on the propensity of the skin to become hyperpigmented caused by an inflammatory stimulus and to sustain that hyperpigmentation for extended periods may prove valuable.

Skin structure differences according to skin color

Reed *et al.* [5] compared the skin structure of subjects with skin types V and VI (4 African Americans, 2 Filipinos, and 1 Hispanic) to those with lightly pigmented skin types II and III (6 Asians and 8 fair skinned subjects.) The darkly pigmented subjects required more tape strippings to disrupt the epidermal barrier. The authors drew two conclusions from this data. First, darkly pigmented skin probably has more cornified cell layers, and therefore is more compact than lightly pigmented skin. Secondly, dark skin is thought to display superior epidermal barrier function. These results are particularly interesting because the differences in cell layers and barrier protection were demonstrated to be related to the skin hue and SPT, not race.

Table 1 demonstrates the main biological differences between dark and fair skinned individuals and the therapeutic implications of those differences.

Development of photoaging in respect to the skin color

Individuals with dark skin are known to have firmer and smoother skin than individuals with lighter skin of the same age [6]. The melanin contents and melanosomal dispersion pattern is thought to confer protection from the accelerated aging induced by exposure to UV radiation. Black epidermis on average provided an SPF of 13.4, which would provide the scientific basis for the "better aging" observation [7]. Photoaging among dark skinned people does occur, but it is more common in individuals with relatively fair skin [6].

Table 1 Therapeutic implications of key biologic differences between dark and fair skinned individuals [1]

Biological Factor	Therapeutic Implications
Epidermis Increased melanin content, melanosomal dispersion in people with dark skin	Lower rates of skin cancer in people of color Less pronounced photoaging
Dermis Multinucleated and larger fibroblasts in dark skinned people compared with fair skinned people	Pigmentation disorders due to both biological predispositions and cultural practices (e.g. use of lightening agents) Greater incidence of keloid formation in black people compared with white people
Hair Curved hair follicle/spiral hair type in black people compared with white people Fewer elastic fibers anchoring hair follicles to dermis in black people compared with white people	Pseudofolliculitis in black people who shave Use of hair products that may lead to hair and scalp disorders in black people Increased incidence of alopecias in black women

Pigmentary disorders

Postinflammatory hyperpigmentation can be considered the default pathophysiologic response to cutaneous injury in people with dark skin. Postinflammatory hyperpigmentation is a common sequelae of acne vulgaris and the acne hyperpigmented macule (AHM) is often the chief complaint in acne patients with skin of color as opposed to the acne per se [8]. These changes should not be construed as trivial cosmetic changes; they can have significant psychological impact in subjects who experience them [9].

Melasma is another pigmentary disorder that occurs frequently in people with dark skin. This disorder is reported to be more prevalent in black, Hispanic, and Asian subjects. Hormonal factors, UV radiation, and the lability of melanocytes are all thought to be contributing etiologic factors [9].

The prevalence of pigmentation disorders in black subjects has resulted in their use of many topical products that are not always prescribed or monitored by physicians. These cultural practices can result in further dermatologic disorders.

Keloidal scar formation

Although keloidal scarring occurs in all races, it is thought to occur much more frequently in people with dark skin [10], ranging from 3 to 18 times more often in people with dark skin compared with fair skinned people. Keloidal scarring develops through a complex and poorly understood interaction between fibroblasts, various cutaneous cells, and cytokines that facilitates the production of excessive collagen and inhibits the degradation of the extracellular matrix components [11]. Research suggests that fibroblasts are larger and binucleated or multinucleated in black people [12]. When thinking about keloidal formation in black skin, it should be noted that the fibroblasts in these individuals are large and numerous with nuclear machinery possibly awaiting stimulus to begin the overproduction of collagen. That stimulus, thought by many to be transforming growth factor beta 1 (TGF-β1) also acts to retard degradation of collagen and other extracellular matrix proteins [11].

Laser treatment in dark skin

Laser therapy has been a mainstay of dermatologic therapy for more than a decade. However, until recently, most published literature focused on the Caucasian patient. The face of the aesthetic patient is changing to be more representative of the ethnic diversity of the world population. To select an appropriate modality, it is imperative that the dermatologic laser surgeon not only be aware of the unique needs of those with darker skin, but also be well versed in laser technology, including the risks and benefits of cutaneous laser procedures as they relate to the specific needs of the ethnic patient [13]. It is important to understand the basic laser principles when treating ethnic and more darkly pigmented skin. The increased melanin content within the epidermis of a more darkly complected individual will interfere with the absorption of laser energy intended for another target, leading to higher risk of problems ranging from increased pain sensation, hypo- or hyperpigmentation of the treated area, up to scarring. The darker skin of ethnic patients is prone to dyschromia and scarring, which are often the reasons these patients initially seek cosmetic consultation. Corrective procedures carry their own risks of dyschromia and scarring, which should be discussed in detail before initiating the laser treatment. Because of the pigmentary changes tendency in darker skin patients, sun exposure and using the sun screens should be an important part of the patient consultation and discussion of the treatment options.

Disorders such as sickle cell anemia, thalassemia, and glucose 6 phosphate dehydrogenase deficiency are more prevalent in African American, Mediterranean, and South-East Asian patients. A detailed medical history should be taken to determine the personal or family history of these hereditary hemolytic diseases that may affect any post-laser healing [13].

LASER INDICATIONS IN DARK SKIN PATIENTS

Benign cutaneous tumors

Laser-resurfacing procedures are effective treatments to smooth benign cutaneous tumors such as syringomas, dermatosis papulosa nigra, and acne keloidalis nuchae, all of which are more prevalent in dark skinned patients. Because of the depth of the lesion, complete removal is unlikely without increased risk of scarring.

The patient must understand that the goal of this procedure is to flatten, smooth, or improve the appearance of the lesion and not completely remove it Fig. 1.

Dermatosis papulosa nigra are benign flesh-colored papules found predominantly on the face, neck, and trunk. Although no treatment is needed, they are often of cosmetic concern and are easily removed through a variety of means including scissor excision, electro-desiccation, and laser ablation or coagulation [13]. When using an ablative laser, one must be careful to use a spot size that does not exceed the diameter of the lesion to minimize risk of collateral thermal damage and hypo or hyperpigmentation of the

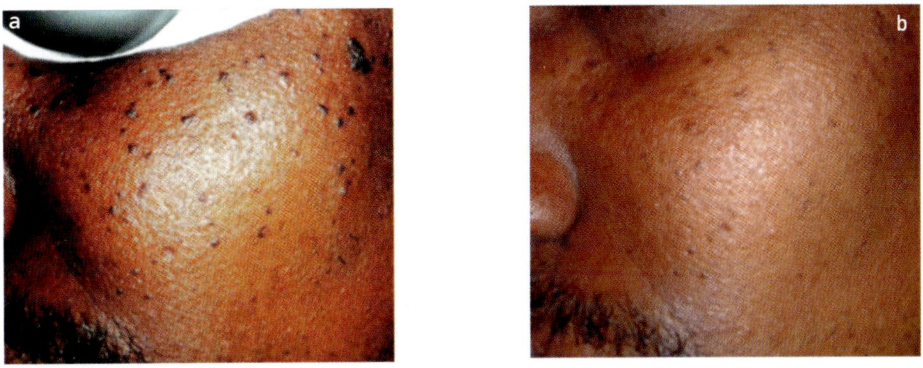

Figure 1 Before laser Nd:YAG treatment emitting at 1,064 nm (a) and 3 weeks after the first session of the treatment of a dermatosis papulosa nigra, without hypo or hyperpigmentation (b)

surrounding skin. **Figure 2** shows temporary hypopigmentation which occurred 1 week after Nd:YAG 1,064 nm laser treatment for DPN in a patient with skin type V. The normal skin pigmentation was restored within 3 weeks.

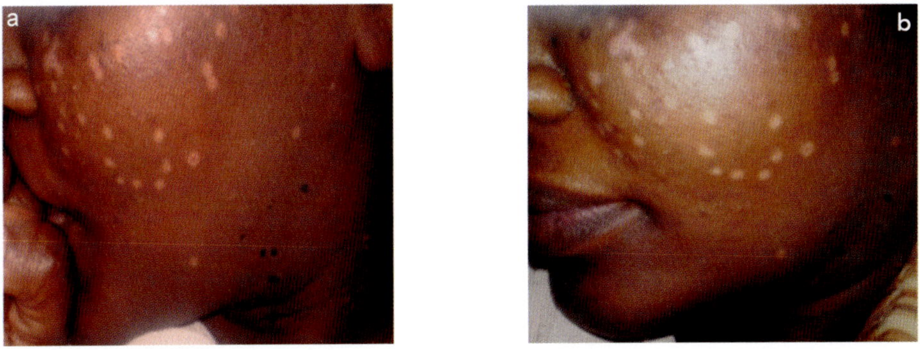

Figure 2 A week after laser Nd:YAG treatment emitting at 1,064 nm on a patient with dermatosis papulosa nigra (a). Hypopigmentation temporarily occurred after the crusts fell (b)

Rhytides and aging skin

Because of the photoprotective nature of melanin in patients with darker skin, crow's feet, smoker's lines, and fine perioral and periorbital lines seen as early as age 20 in the Caucasian patient tend to occur much later, if at all, in patients with darker skin.

Patients with darker skin tend to manifest signs of aging in the deeper muscular layers of the face, with sagging of the malar fat pads toward the nasolabial folds [14].

CONCLUSION

When performing laser procedures in patients with darker skin, the physician's challenge of optimal treatment lies in the ability to balance effective treatment with minimal risk to the patient. Untoward effects may be minimized with the use of conservative treatment parameters and lower energy settings in dark skin. Cutaneous laser surgery has been a mainstay of dermatologic therapy for more than a decade; however, until recently, most published studies have excluded patients with darker skin. With appropriate patient selection and proper physician training, laser surgery is increasingly safe in patients with dark skin.

REFERENCES

[1] Taylor S. Skin of color: Biology, structure, function, and implications for dermatologic disease. J Am Acad Dermatol 2002; 46: S41-S62.
[2] Fitzpatrick TB. The validity and practicality of sun reactive skin type I through VI. Arch Dermatol 1988; 124: 869-871.
[3] Pathak MA, Nghiem P, Fitzpatrick TB. Acute and chronic effects of the sun. In: Freedberg IM, Eisen AZ, Wolff K, Austen KF, Goldsmith LA, Katz SI, *et al.*, editors. Fitzpatrick's dermatology in general medicine, vol. 1. New York (NY): McGraw-Hill; 1999, p. 1598-1608.
[4] Lancer HA. Lancer Ethnicity Scale (LES) [correspondence]. Lasers Surg Med 1998; 22: 9.
[5] Reed JT, Ghadially R, Elias PM. Effect of race gender, and skin type of epidermal permeability barrier function [abstract]. J Invest Dermatol 1994; 102: 537.
[6] Halder RM. The role of retinoids in the management of Cutaneous conditions in blacks. J Am Acad Dermatol 1998; 39: S98-S103.
[7] Kaidbey KH, Agin PP, Sayre RM, Kligman A. Photoprotection by melanin-a comparison of black and caucasian skin. J Am Acad Dermatol 1979; 1: 249-260.
[8] Cress RD, Holly EA. Incidence of cutaneous melanoma among non-Hispanic whites, Hispanics, Asians, and blacks: an analysis of California Cancer Registry data, 1988-93. Cancer Causes Control 1997; 8: 246-252.
[9] Grimes PE, Stockton T. Pigmentary disorders in blacks. Dermatol Clin 1988; 6: 271-281.
[10] Ketchum LD, Cohen IK, Masters FW. Hypertrophic scars and keloidal scars. Plast Reconstr Surg 1974; 53: 140-154.
[11] Johnson BL Jr. Keloids. In: Johnson BL Jr, Moy RL, White GM, editors. Ethnic skin: medical and surgical. St. Louis (MO): Mosby; 1998, p. 167-170.
[12] Montagna W, Carlisle K. The architecture of black and white facial skin. J Am Acad Dermatol 1991; 24: 929-937.
[13] Jackson B. Lasers in ethnic skin: A review. J Am Acad Dermatol 2003; 48: S134-S138.
[14] Matory WE. Aging in people of color. In: Matory WE, editor. Ethnic considerations in facial aesthetic surgery. Philadelphia (PA): Lippincott-Raven; 1998, p. 151-170.

CHAPTER 18

Lasers and North African skin

Laila Benzekri

INTRODUCTION

In North Africa, just as in Europe, there has been a growing enthusiasm for corrective dermatology using lasers for a number of years. In this chapter, after defining the specific ethnic features of the population requesting treatment, we will discuss in turn: the specific reasons for requesting treatment and the most commonly upheld indications and types of laser used, the treatment protocols offered, the side effects reported, and the preventive steps to be taken according to the phototype, the strong sunlight, and the dressing customs and rituals.

North African phototypes and their impact on pathophysiology and treatment

In North Africa, all phototypes can be seen: the light phototypes I, II and III of the Berber and Andalusian populations (blond or red hair and light eyes), the darker phototype IV, which is in the majority, the black-skinned phototypes V and much more rarely VI. This ethnic diversity in skin colour is determined in several ways: genetically, biochemically, and cytologically in terms of the type of melanin produced but also with regard to the ability of keratinocytes to destroy the melanin that is inappropriately produced for the season.

It is easy to understand that genetic diversity has an effect on which type of melanin is produced, on the structure of the melanosome protein skeleton, and on what happens to melanin within the keratinocytes. A reasoned assessment of all these phenomena should lead to a reduction in therapeutic transgressions in terms of post-treatment pigmentary side effects.

Nature of melanin produced according to phototype

Melanocytes are capable of producing both sulfur-containing pheomelanin and black eumelanin [1-7]. At the extreme ends of the spectrum, the melanocytes of subjects with the light skin phototypes I and II mainly produce pheomelanin and those of the black-skinned phototype V produce mainly eumelanin.

Between the two, the melanocytes in phototypes III and IV produce a mixture of pheomelanin and eumelanin with the pheomelanin/eumelanin ratio tipping as the subject's phototype gets closer along the spectrum to V [8, 2, 9]. Post-treatment pigmentary side effects will be more common in subjects who have a higher phototype (with eumelanin) and practically non-existent in those who have light phototypes (with pheomelanin).

Melanosome protein skeleton structure

Melanosomes of increased size that are individually distributed will be more difficult for enzymes from lysosome vacuoles to digest. At the extreme end, the melanosomes in black skin, which are sometimes larger than 1μ, will not be destroyed and will be eliminated into the stratum corneum. This is how we conclude that unseasonal hyperpigmentation depends not only on phototype but also on the epidermal unit as a whole with both melanocytes and keratinocytes being of equal importance [9, 10].

Outcome of melanin in keratinocytes

The genetic control of skin colour involves not only the production of melanin, but also the autophagy of melanin by keratinocytes [4]. This basic notion has a tendency to be misunderstood and it must be taken into account [11]. Indeed, the ethnic diversity of skin colour is basically due to the regulation of melanin degradation by epidermal keratinocytes [4]. Small melanosomes carrying pheomelanin or eumelanin will easily be destroyed and will not lead to pigmentary side effects. By contrast, large melanosomes carrying eumelanin will be difficult to destroy and will accumulate in the epidermis leading to relatively long-lasting hyperpigmentation. In the absence of a signal to trigger melanogenesis (UV or inflammatory factors), the preventive use of hydroquinone, which acts as a sort of decoy due to its molecular similarity to tyrosine, has no scientific justification and is purely speculative.

MANAGING PATIENTS WITH VARIED PHOTOTYPES

In our management of patients with varied phototypes, we try to take these basic pathophysiological concepts into account.

Dermatological lasers: patients' specific requests, suitable indications

On its website, the French Dermatology Society (Société Française de Dermatologie) has validated the following as being indications suitable for management with dermatological lasers: broken capillaries, some kinds of angioma, varicose veins [9], some types of hyperpigmentation, tattoo removal, hirsutism, scars, skin aging, etc. We must adjust these treatments to suit the phototypes encountered in North Africa.

Specific requests made by patients living in North Africa

Patients mainly wish to undergo laser correction for cosmetic hair removal, hirsutism, acne scars, skin aging, rosacea, spider angiomas, vascular naevi, lentigines, tattoo removal, varicose veins, and cellulite.

Suitable indications

It is clear that there sometimes is a gap between some patients' requests, which are refused (such as waxing downy hair), and the indications that are ultimately upheld. They broadly correspond to the requests made by the patients. The treatment of ingrown hair in men or women is a common indication in darker phototypes for the use of hair removal lasers.

Management

During the first consultation, the patient is informed of what results can be expected, the structure and duration of the treatment, the possible side effects and how to prevent them, as well as the cost the treatment. Medical history will be examined to include dermatological and other events, and any current medical treatment that could be a contraindication to treatment with dermatological lasers. Previous disappointing results or failed treatments with lasers (with the type of laser to be specified) will be taken into consideration. In addition, we try to answer any questions that the patient might have. A later meeting will be scheduled so the patient has time to think about it. Further laboratory tests will be carried out if the patient is consulting for hirsutism or lower limb varicose veins.

Choice of laser

It is clear that the choice of laser depends on the abnormality to be corrected [12], the phototype, and the selection of lasers available. For example, non-ablative wavelengths are a good choice for initiating treatment of acne scars in dark skin [13]. For rejuvenation, there is minimal literature focusing on the laser resurfacing of dark phototypes [14, 5]. Research is necessary to determine the non-ablative and ablative wavelengths that produce the best results and, most importantly, avoid complications.

For hypertrichosis or laser hair removal in dark skins, 800 nm laser diodes and the 1,064 nm Nd:YAG laser are used more widely than alexandrite lasers, which should be used with caution. This is because these systems offer lower melanin absorption.

For tattoo removal, the methodology varies depending on whether the tattoo was performed as part of a ritual, by an amateur, or a professional. We see fewer and fewer traditional tattoos and an increasing numbers of amateur and professional tattoos. Q-switched and Nd:YAG lasers (which we use most often) and alexandrite lasers produce good results with few side effects or incidences of post-operative hyperpigmentation. Traditional or ritual tattoos, which are black or more often blue, can be treated quickly and more effectively than professional tattoos.

In terms of vascular lasers, while pulsed dye lasers or KTP lasers can be used in light phototypes, use of a Nd:YAG laser is preferred in darker skin because of the risk of dyschromia.

Methodology for use of various lasers in dark phototypes

The methodology depends on the laser used, the type and extent of abnormality to be corrected, and the environmental and occupational conditions of the patient [6, 15, 16].

Fluence: start with low fluences and use a long pulse duration then gradually increase the fluence using a shorter pulse duration. Based on the results observed, the optimal fluence parameter can be determined.

Test: in darker phototypes, between two and four fluences are tested to determine the ideal fluence and assess the risk of side effects.

Scheduling of sessions: laser treatments will be stopped during periods of full sunshine, at their peak during the summer. However, use of a Nd:YAG laser for hair removal can continue all year round without interruption. In practice, the interval between sessions depends on the laser being used and the abnormality being treated: 1 month for hair removal lasers, 2-3 months for vascular lasers, 2 months for tattoo removal, 1.5 months for rejuvenation in fair skins and 2 months for rejuvenation in dark skins.

Side effects and prevention [17]

Infection: bacterial infections are very rare as long as the rules of pre- and post-operative asepsis are followed.

Preventing post-laser scars and burns: high fluences should be avoided. We use healing, soothing, and hydrating creams until the treated area has healed to avoid crusts forming. Hypertrophic and keloid scars are a risk in darker phototypes.

Pigmentary side effects: care is essential when treating glabrous skin because it does not have “emergency” melanocyte reservoirs to intervene in post-operative repigmentation. Similarly, to avoid permanent depigmentation, high fluences should be avoided. A short course of moderately potent topical corticosteroids (desonide, hydrocortisone aceponate, etc.) will control the post-epilatory inflammatory phenomena that could potentially lead to hyperpigmentation.

Preventing side effects

Herpes prevention: a prescription of valaciclovir is offered in treatment with fractional ablative lasers for patients with recurrent outbreaks or a history of herpes infection.

Sun protection: protection from the sun involving application of sunscreens begins before a session of alexandrite laser and continues afterwards, over 15-30 days for hair removal lasers. After treatment with fractional ablative and non-ablative lasers and vascular lasers, sun protection should be maintained for at least six months. In addition to the use of topical sun protection, it is useful to wear clothes offering coverage, hats, and sunglasses.

Modulation and control of post-treatment inflammatory reaction: topical corticosteroids are prescribed for two to three days until red blotches disappear after treatment with hair removal lasers.

Make-up: the application of scented make-up and essential oils to the area to be treated must be avoided on the day of the laser treatment, since the skin must be thoroughly cleaned. By contrast, the use of make-up to correct the complexion after laser treatment is permitted. Visits to swimming pools or steam rooms are not advisable until healing is complete.

After hair removal lasers: paradoxical hypertrichosis is often seen in our practice as it is in other Mediterranean countries. In an unpublished Moroccan study of 601 females, 3.16% of patients presented paradoxical hypertrichosis within 5-35 months. To prevent this, two passes with the Nd:YAG laser were routinely performed, focusing on the edges of the area to be treated and especially the face. Another option is to cool the treated area immediately after the laser treatment.

CONCLUSION

Management using dermatological lasers in North Africa does not depend solely on the phototypes of patients, which are very varied in the final analysis, but more on the environmental conditions and especially the constant presence of the sun over many months of the year. A strict patient selection process and choice of treatment date, as well as a careful choice of the laser to be used, should reduce the risk of side effects in patients with dark phototypes. It is worth noting that these patients are less likely to present photoaging lesions than subjects with light phototypes.

REFERENCES

[1] Inazu M, Mishima Y. Detection of eumelanogenic and pheomelanogenic melanosomes in the same normal human melanocyte. J Invest Dermatol 1993; 100: 172S-175S.

[2] Jimbow K. N-Acetyl -4-S Cysteaminyl phenol as a new type of depigmenting agent for the melanoderma patients with melasma. Arch Dermatol 1991; 127 (10): 1528-1534.

[3] Loo WJ, Lanigan SW. Recent advances in laser therapy for the treatment of cutaneous vascular disorders. Lasers Med Sci 2002; 17 (1): 9-11.

[4] Murase D, Hachya A, Takano K, Hicks R, Visscher MO, *et al.* Authophagy has a significant role in determining skin color by regulating melanosome degradation in keratinocytes. J Invest Dermatol 2013; 165: 1-9.

[5] Ruiz-Esparza J, Barba Gomez JM, Gomez de la Torre OL, Huerta Franco B, Parga Vazquez EG. UltraPulse laser skin resurfacing in Hispanic patients. A prospective study of 36 individuals. Dermatol Surg 1998; 24: 59-62.

[6] Shah S, Alster P. Laser treatment of dark skin: an updated review. Am J Clin Dermatol. 2010; 11(6): 389-397.

[7] Smit NP, Van der Meulen H, Koertin HK, Kolb RM, Pavel S. Melanogenesis in cultured melanocytes can be substantially influenced by L Tyrosine and L Cysteine. J Invest Dermatol 1997; 109: 796-800.
[8] Alaluf S, Atkins D, Barrett K, Blount M, Carter N, Heath A. Ethnic variation in melanin content and composition in photoexposed and photoprotected human skin. Pigment Cell Res 2002; 15: 112-118.
[9] Tadokoro T, Yamaguchi Y, Batzer J, *et al.* Mechanisms of skin tanning in different racial/ethnic groups in response to ultraviolet radiation. J Invest Dermatol 2005; 124: 1326-1332.
[10] Van Niewport FV, Smit FM, Kolb R, Van der Meulen H, Koertin H, Pavel S. Tyrosine-induced melanogenesis shows differences in morphologic and melanogenesis preferences of melanosomes from light and dark skin types. J Invest Dermatol 2004; 122 (5): 1251-1255.
[11] Though Y, Jee SE, Sun CC, Boissy RE. The patterns of melanosomes distribution in keratinocytes of human skin as one determining factor of skin colour. Br J Dermatol 2008; 149: 498-505.
[12] Anderson J. Lasers in dermatology: a critical update. J Dermatol 2000; 27 (11): 700-705.
[13] Taylor SC, Cook-Bolden F, Rahman Z, Strachan D. Acne vulgaris in skin of color. J Am Acad Dermatol 2002; 46 (2, Suppl): S98-S106.
[14] Goh CL, Khoo L. Laser skin resurfacing treatment outcome of facial scars and wrinkles in Asians with skin type III/IV with the Unipulse CO_2 laser system. Singapore Med J 2002; 43: 28-32.
[15] Bhatt N, Alster TS. Laser surgery in dark skin. Dermatol Surg 2008; 34: 184-194, discussion 194-195.
[16] Cole PD, Hatef DA, Kaufman Y, Jason N. Lasertherapy in ethnic populations. Semin Plast Surg 2009; 23(3): 173-177.
[17] Haedersdal M. Cutaneous side effects from laser treatment of the skin. Acta Der Venereol 1999; 207: 1-32.

Conclusion

The management of facial skin aging or facial rejuvenation involves a specialised consultation, in which the dermatologist's expertise is the foundation for the choice of a treatment program aiming to reach a consensus over the objectives to be achieved: a satisfactory result for both the doctor and the patient.

Injections using botulinum toxin and dermal fillers are currently the most commonly used techniques worldwide and most of the time they produce satisfactory results, but they do require maintenance sessions at regular intervals, and their use is limited to their respective field of indications.

The results, obtained using these techniques, do not lead to improvements in the epidermal changes caused by aging and aggravated by the consequences of exposure to the sun or dermatoheliosis. The same holds true for cutaneous laxity: a relatively deep deterioration of the dermis, it is a consequence of extremely variable intrinsic aging processes, and depends on each individual's genetics and numerous environmental and lifestyle factors.

Lasers and EBD provide an answer to these problems, albeit an imperfect one. The aesthetic issues related to skin aging constitute the motives of the patients seeking consultations with practitioners who dedicate a sizeable part of their practice to such problems.

This consultation remains above all, in our eyes, a medical one, during which a consensus needs to be reached between the doctor and the patient: one or several techniques must be chosen; unrealistic expectations must be avoided; information must be provided about alternative techniques such as plastic and reconstructive surgery.

The patient will be offered a holistic and personalised treatment plan, in which treatments using lasers and EBD may be combined with injections of toxin products, dermal fillers, or peels, following a specified schedule.

There is a plethora of techniques and it is difficult for a layperson, or even for an experienced doctor, to select a treatment from the multitude of options available. The main purpose of this work is to assist our readers in making this choice. Our work represents the most exhaustive analysis possible of innovative technologies from international experts with an aim to provide the greatest consensual and shared openness.

We would like to particularly thank the authors, especially those from outside Europe, who have agreed to share their knowledge, their expertise, and their daily experience, which is already equivalent to ours due to the globalisation of people and economies.

It is our hope that this book will remain "open" for any questions you may have today, and even to a future edition.

Serge Dahan, Bertrand Pusel

Annexes Iconography

CO_2 RESURFACING

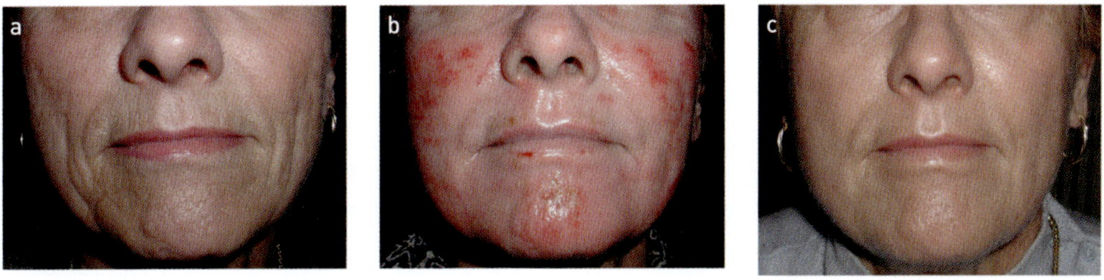

Figure 1 Before treatment (a), 7 days after (b) and 60 days after 1 session of CO_2 ultrapulsed laser treatment (c)
(photos S. Angel)

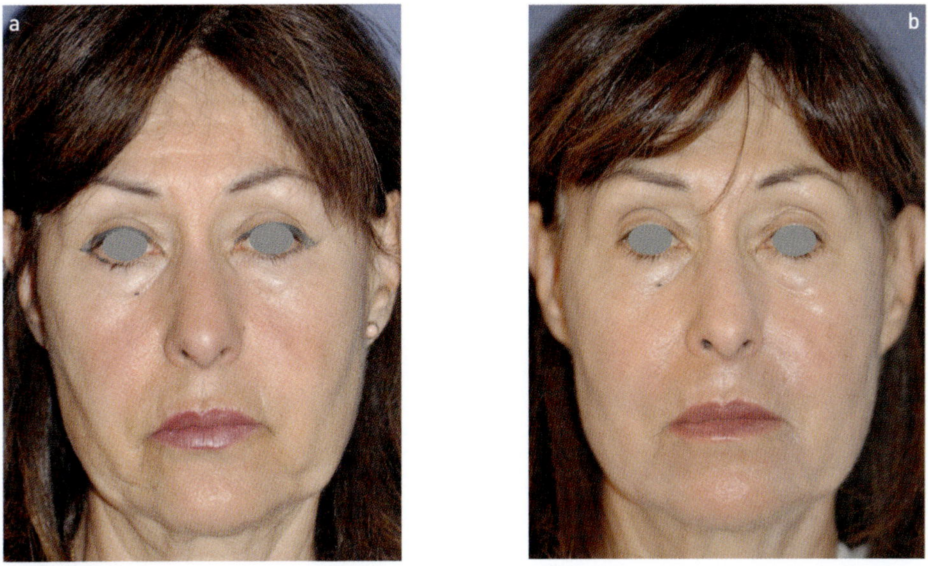

Figure 2 Belfore (a) and 3 months after one session of CO_2 SmartXide DOT^2 laser treatment (b)
Result: Note the effect on laxity on the oval and the lower part of the face
(photos A. Le Pillouer-Prost)

CO_2 FRACTIONAL ABLATIVE LASER

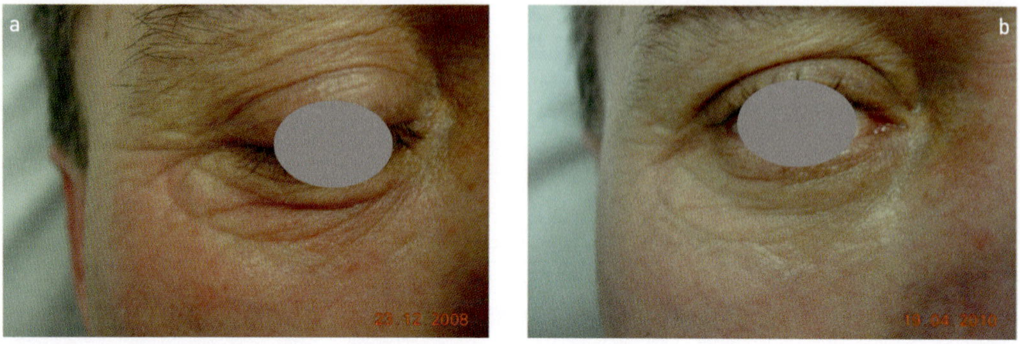

Figure 3 Before (a) and after 3 sessions of CO_2 fractional laser treatment (b)
(photos R. Bousquet-Rouaud)

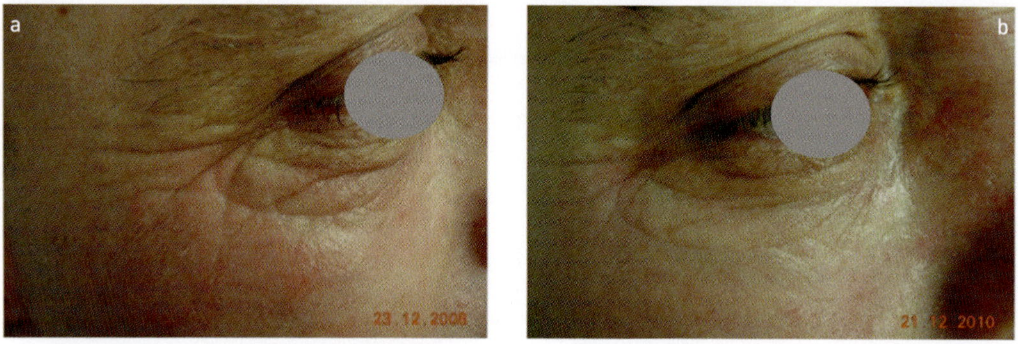

Figure 4 Before CO_2 fractional laser treatment (a) and result 2 years after (b)
(photos R. Bousquet-Rouaud)

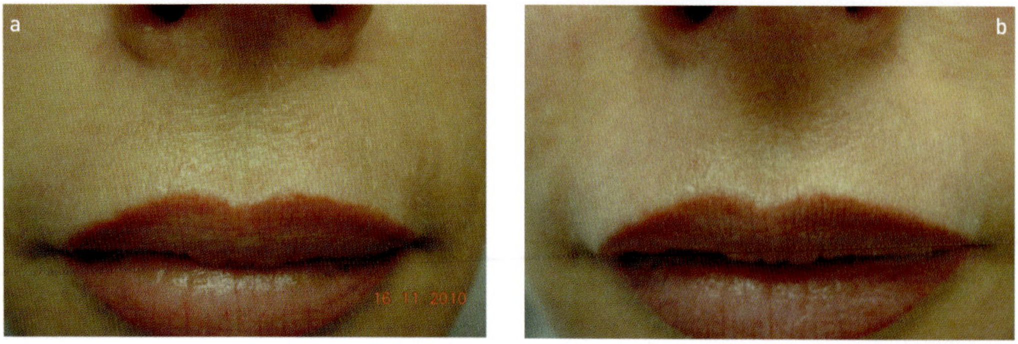

Figure 5 Before (a) and 3 months after 1 session of CO_2 fractional laser treatment (b)
(photos R. Bousquet-Rouaud)

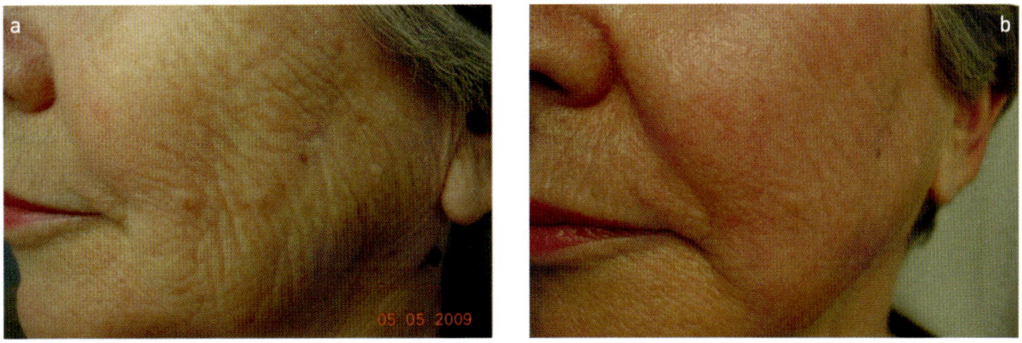

Figure 6 Before (a) and after 3 sessions of fractional CO_2 laser treatment (b)
(photos R. Bousquet-Rouaud)

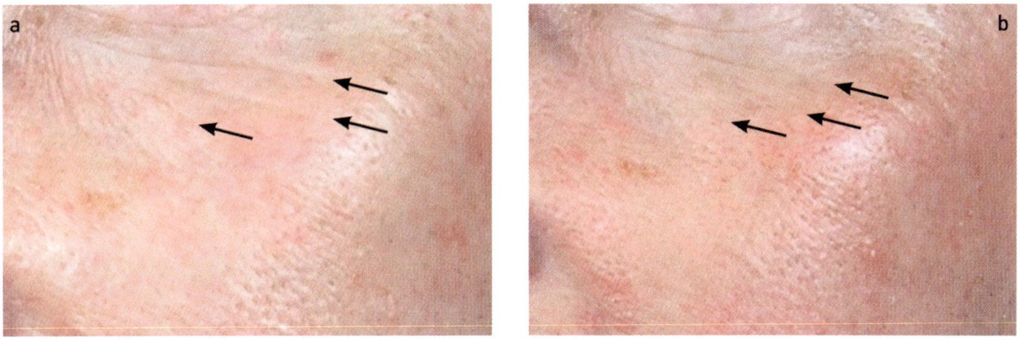

Figure 7 Before (a) and 3 months after 2 sessions of fractional CO_2 laser treatment (b)
(photos S. Angel)

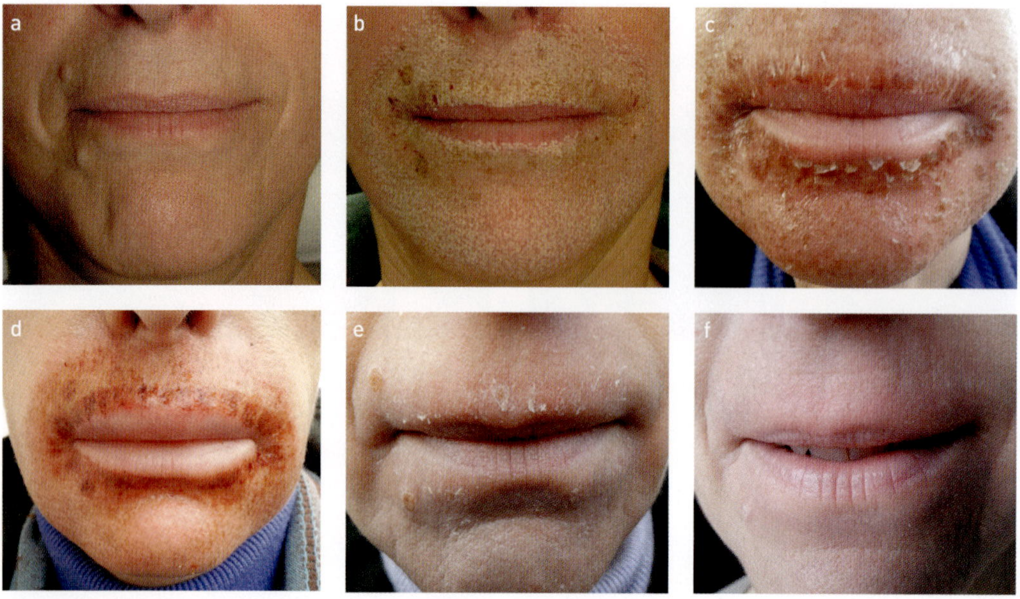

Figure 8 Before treatment (a), after 1 session of fractional CO_2 laser treatment (b)
Scarring at day 2 (c), 5 (d) and 7 (e) and result three months later (f)
(photos H. Cartier)

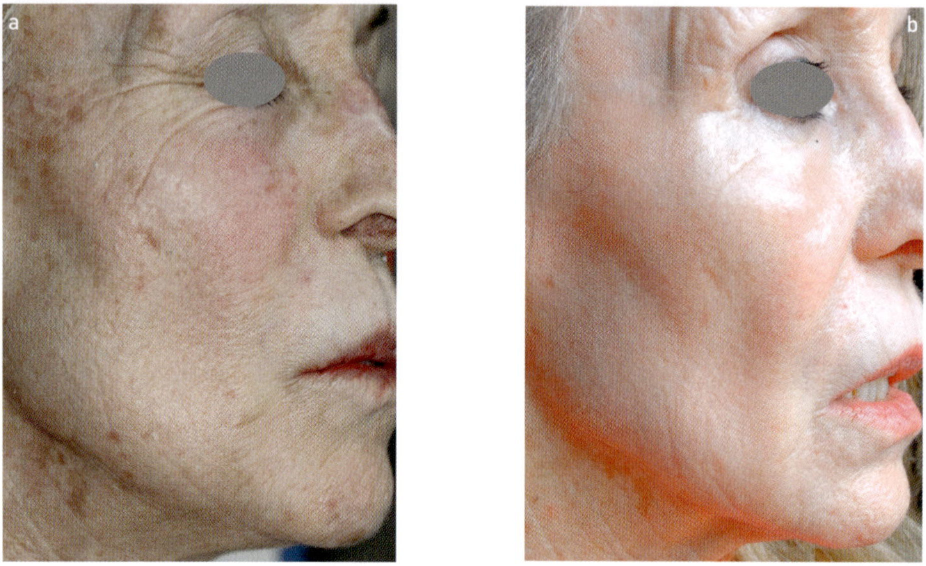

Figure 9 Before treatment (a) and one month after a session of fractional CO_2 laser treatment (b)
(photos T. Passeron)

NON ABLATIVE FRACTIONAL LASER

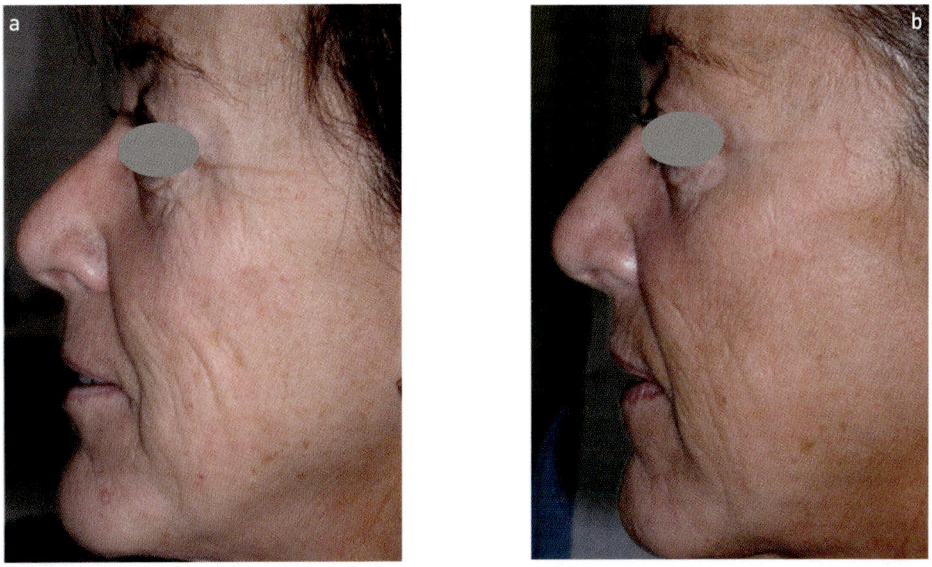

Figure 10 Before treatment (a) and 3 months after 3 sessions of non ablative fractional laser (1,550 nm) treatment (b)
(photos B. Pusel)

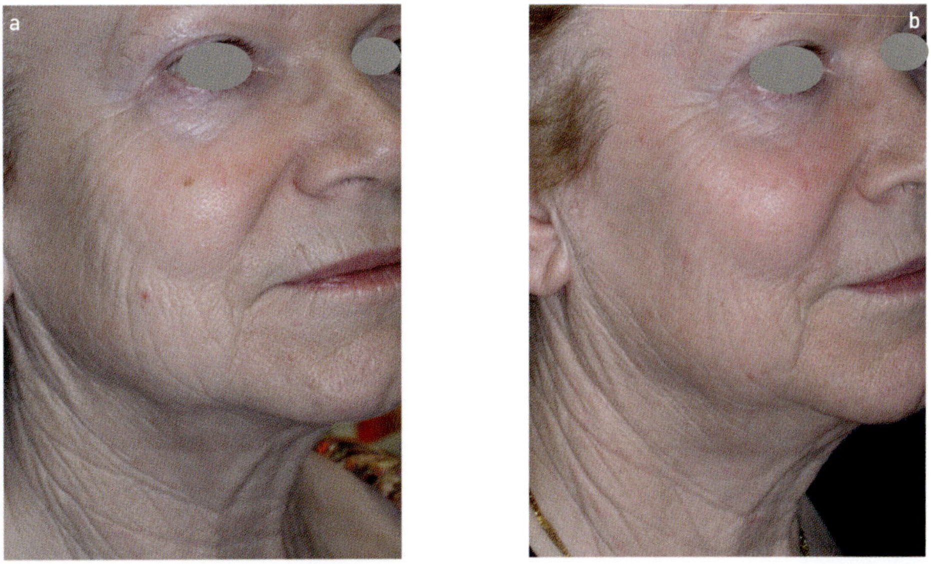

Figure 11 Before treatment (a) and 3 months after 3 sessions of non ablative fractional laser (1,550 nm) treatment (b)
(photos B. Pusel)

MONOPOLAR RADIOFREQUENCY

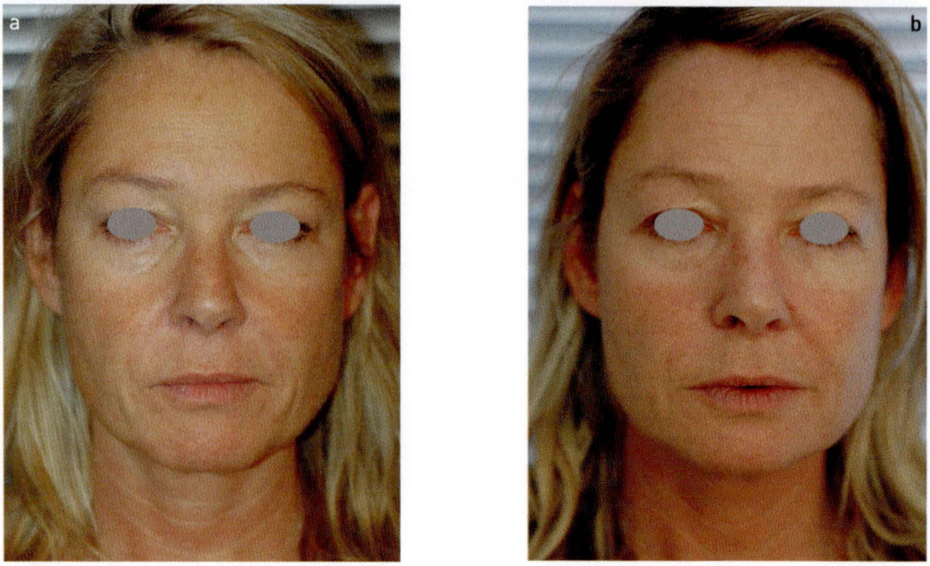

Figure 12 Before (a) and after 4 months of monopolar radiofrequency treatment (b) *(photos M. Magis)*

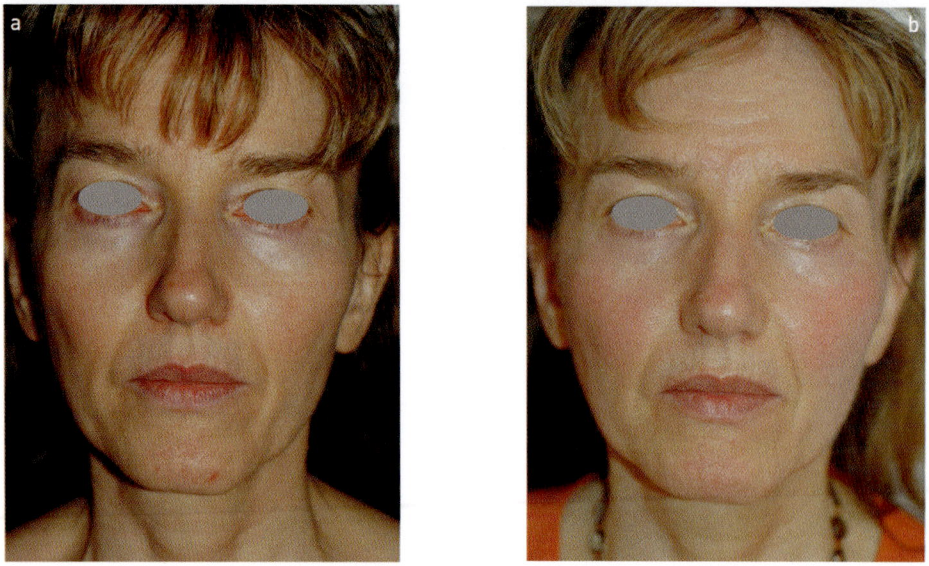

Figure 13 Before (a) and after one year of monopolar radiofrequency treatment (b) *(photos M. Magis)*

BIPOLAR RADIOFREQUENCY

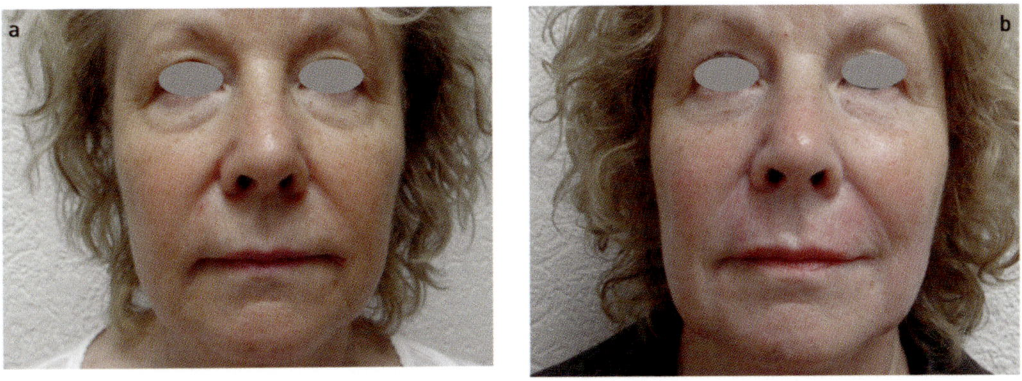

Figure 14 Before (a) and after 3 years of bipolar radiofrequency treatment: 1 session per month during 6 months and then 1 session every 3 months during 4 months (b)
(photos I. Rousseaux)

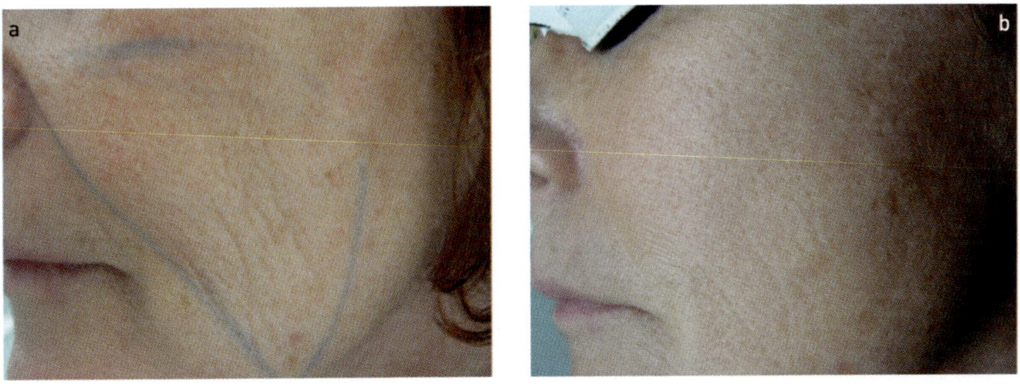

Figure 15 Before (a) and after fractional radiofrequency treatment: good efficacy on the cheeks (b)
(photos S. Dahan)

LASER Q-SWITCHED

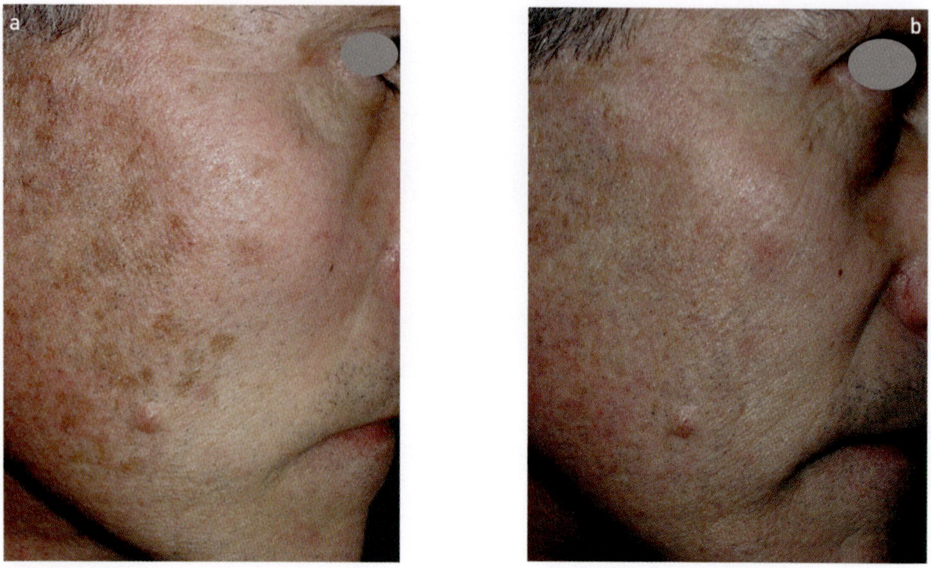

Figure 16 Actinic keratosis before (a) and one month after QSY 532 nm 1.8 J/cm^2 laser treatment (b)
(photos M. Magis)

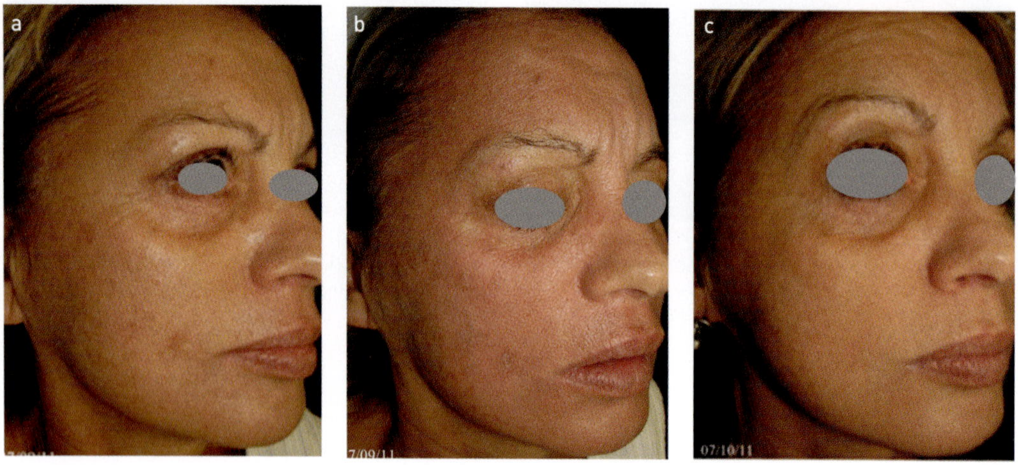

Figure 17 Before photorejuvenation by QSY 532 nm laser only (a), sun burn effect of peeling-QSY 532 nm laser (b), lightening of the skin tone and erasal of lentigos, with homogenous skin tone ten days after 1 QSY laser session (c)
(photos H. Cartier)

COMBINED TREATMENTS: LASER CO_2 + Q-SWITCHED LASER

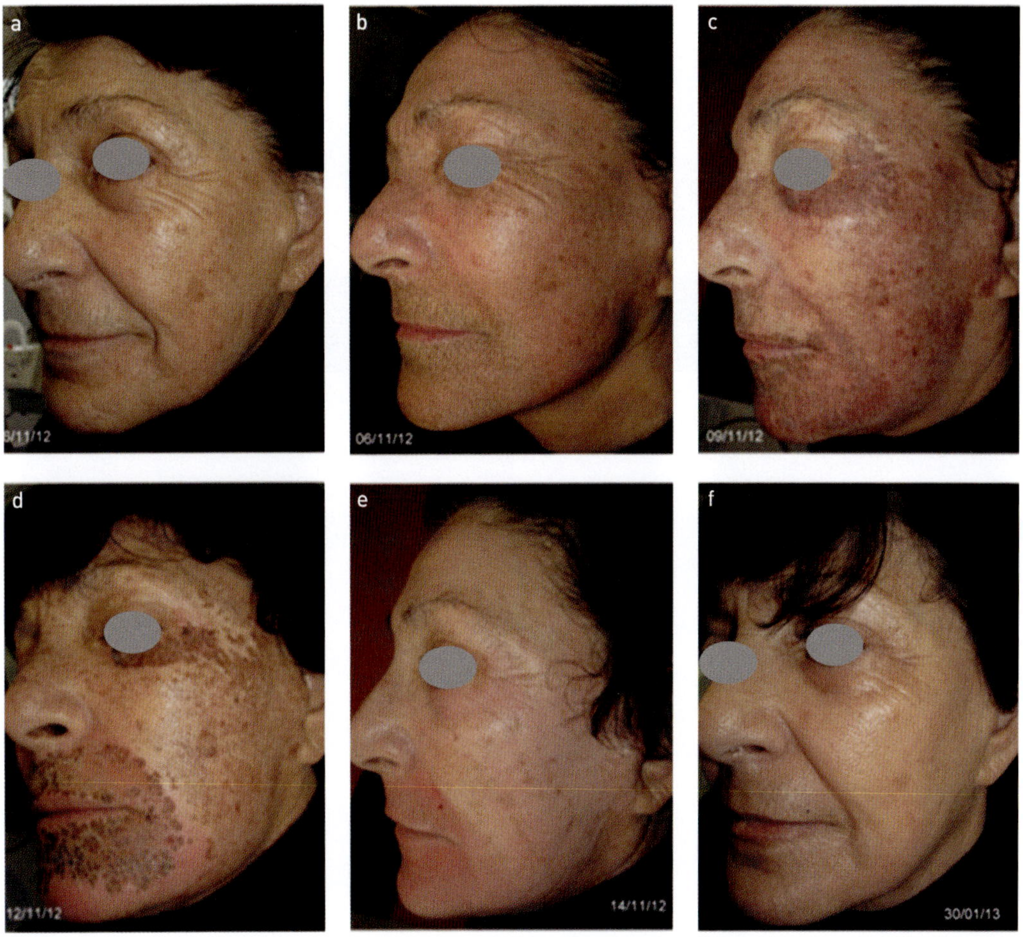

Figure 18 Advanced heliodermis associating wrinkles and lentigos (a), immediately after fractional CO_2 laser on the month and eye zone and remodeling by QSY 1,064 nm laser, followed by QSY 532 nm laser-peeling (b), scarring phase at days 3 (c), disintegration of crusts at day 6, those on CO_2 laser treated areas being longer to heal (d), final epidermisation phase with post-laser erythema at day 14 (e), final result: homogenous and global rejuvenation of the face with one session of fractional CO_2 laser around the mouth and eyes, and QSY laser on the other areas of the face (f)
(photos H. Cartier)

COMBINED TREATMENTS: PULSED LIGHT + BIPOLAR RADIOFREQUENCY + FRACTIONAL RADIOFREQUENCY

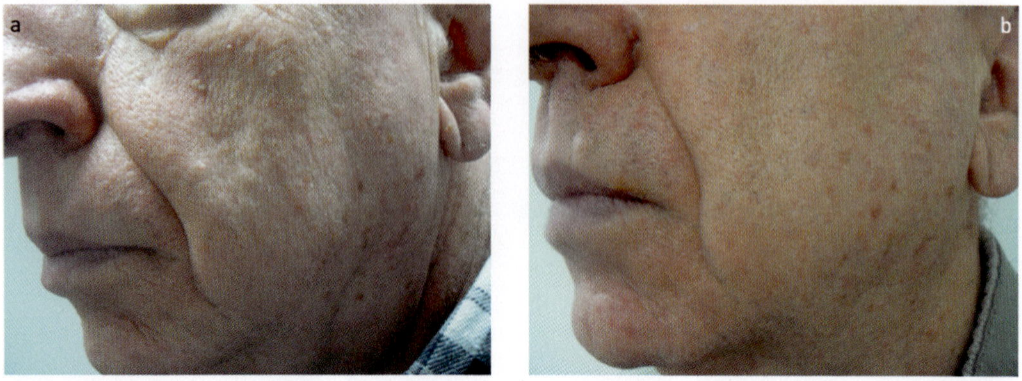

Figure 19 Before (a) and after treatment by pulsed light, bipolar radiofrequency + fractional radiofrequency *(photos S. Dahan)*

IMPRIM'VERT®

Achevé d'imprimer par Corlet, Imprimeur, S.A.
14110 Condé-sur-Noireau
N° d'Imprimeur : 164366 - Dépôt légal : septembre 2014
Imprimé en France